BREVILLE AIR FRYER OVEN COOKBOOK:

250 Quick and Flavorful Recipes to Cook Fast & Healthy Meals for You and Your Family (Including Vegetarian and Vegan Options)

Table of Contents

Introduction

The Breville Smart Air Fryer Oven is a conducive way to cook appetizing healthy meals. The machine makes use of fast, hot air to cook the food. This allows the outside of the food to be crisp and also ensures that the inner layers are cooked.

The fryer allows us to cook almost everything and many dishes. We can use the deep fryer for cooking meat, vegetables, poultry, fruits, fish, and a wide variety of desserts.

How does the fryer work?

The innovation of the fryer is very easy and simple. Fried foods have a crisp texture because the hot oil heats the food quickly and equally on its surface. Oil is an excellent conductor of heat, which helps to cook all the ingredients quickly and simultaneously.

For decades, chefs have used transfer ovens to mimic the effects of frying or cooking across the entire surface of the food. But the air never revolves fast enough to achieve this wonderful crunchy surface that we all enjoy in fried foods.

With this process, the air circulates in high degrees, up to 201 ° C, to "fry" any food such as chicken, fish, or chips, etc. This innovation has changed the whole idea of cooking by reducing fat by up to 80% compared to traditional fried fat. Cooking the deep fryer releases heat through a heating element that cooks food in a healthier and more convenient way.

There is also an exhaust fan just above the cooking chamber that provides the necessary airflow for the food. In this way, the food is prepared with constant hot air. This leads to the same heating temperature that reaches each part of the food that is cooked. Therefore, only the grill and exhaust fan helps the fryer to propel the air at a constant high speed to cook healthy food with less fat.

Internal pressure increases the temperature, which is then controlled by the exhaust system. The extractor fan also releases additional filtered air to cook food in a much healthier way. The deep fryer does not smell at all and is completely harmless, making it easy to use and environmentally friendly.

Benefits of the deep fryer

Healthier meals without oil

- Eliminate kitchen odors using internal air filters

- Facilitates cleaning due to lack of lubricating oils

- Air Fryers can bake, bake, broil and fry, providing more options.

- Has the ability to adjust and exit from most models and includes a digital timer

The fryer is all-in-one that allows for quick and easy cooking. It also leads to many possibilities once you know it. Once you know the basics and become familiar with your fryer, you can experiment and modify the recipes in any way you prefer. You can prepare a large number of dishes in the fryer and customize your favorite oven to be compatible with the fryer. Everything comes in variety and many options, right?

Cooking perfect, delicious, and healthy meals have never been easier. You can see how this collection of recipes looks.

Enjoy!

CHAPTER 1:

Understanding Breville Smart Air Fryer Oven

Breville Smart Air Fryer Oven

The Breville Smart Fryer is among the smart appliances for cooking and cooking. It looks like a transfer oven and also fries or cooks your food using the transfer method. The hot air revolves around the food placed on the cooking tray. The heating elements are displayed on the top of the Breville Smart Deep Fryer with a full power fan. The fan aids to circulate the hot air flow evenly in the oven. This will allow you to cook your food quickly and evenly on all sides. Fry your food in much less oil. Take a tablespoon or less than a tablespoon of oil to fry and mash your food.

The Breville Smart Fryer is not only used to fry your food, but also to grill your favorite chicken, bake cakes and cookies, and also reheat your frozen foods. It comes with 13 smart cooking modes. These functions are toast, muffin, bake, broil, broil, pizza, cookies, warm, hot, potato, waterproof, dehydrated, and slow cook. It works with an intelligent Element IQ system that finds the cold spot and automatically adjusts the temperature with PID temperature sensing and the digital control, giving you even and accurate cooking. The smart fryer oven works with double speed transfer technology; with this technique, you can cook your food faster by reducing cooking time by transferring. The smart fryer comes with a display that shows the 11 smart functions, as well as the cooking temperature and time. The smart fryer is also equipped with a built-in oven light, you can turn this light on at any time to see the cooking progress, or it can turn on automatically after the cook cycle is complete.

The Smart Deep Fryer is made from the most durable materials. The oven shell is made of reinforced stainless steel. In the smart oven, quartz is used instead of the metallic element because the quartz responds faster compared to the metallic element. Heat your oven quickly and evenly. The interior of the smart oven is lined with a non-stick coating that makes your daily cleaning process easy. To avoid burns, the oven rack is a self-extracting magnetic shelf. When you open the oven door, the shelves are automatically removed in the middle of the oven.

The Breville Smart Oven Fryer has one of the most flexible cooking appliances that are easy for everyone to handle. It is more than just a toaster that functions as a deep fryer, working pot, slow cooker, and also has the ability to dehydrate food. If air frying alone is not your main goal, this is the right choice for your kitchen. This smart oven works very well to heat food to the right temperature thanks to the transfer technology. It is one of the more expensive toaster ovens in this section. If your main concern is more function, good performance, and flexibility, then the Breville Smart Oven Fryer is the best choice for your family.

How to Prepare the Smart Oven before the First Use

It is necessary to empty the smart oven for 20 minutes before the first use to remove any protective substance adhering to the elements. Before testing, first, place your oven in a well-ventilated area and follow the instructions below.

1. First, remove the advertising stickers, multiple covers, or any packing material from the oven.

2. Remove the baking sheet, crumb tray, dehydrator basket or skillet, pizza tray, baking sheet, broil rack, multi-pack rack, and wash in hot water or soapy water with a cloth smooth and pat dry.

3. Take a soft, damp sponge to clean the inside of the oven and dry it well.

4. Place your oven in a well-ventilated area, making sure it is at least 4-6 inches apart on both sides of the oven.

5. Place the crumb tray into the oven in place and plug the power cord into an electrical outlet.

6. The oven display will illuminate with an alarm sound, and the function menu will appear, and the default display is in the TOAST menu setting.

7. Now turn the SELECT / CONFIRM dial until the pointer reaches the PIZZA setting.

8. Press the START / STOP button. After pressing this button, the button's backlight glows red, and the digital oven display glows orange with an audible alert.

9. The display shows the heating flashing. After healing is complete, the oven alarms and timer automatically start measurements.

10. After completing the beeping oven cycle warning, turn off the START / STOP backlight, and the oven LCD display will turn white. This will indicate that the oven is ready for its first use.

Smart Oven Air Fryer Features

Breville smart air fryer comes with 13 smart cooking functions. These functions are as follows

1. TOAST: This function is used to toast the bread. Makes your bread brown and crisp on the outside.

2. BAGEL: This function is used to crisp the inside of the cut bun and also to make light toast on the outside. It is also ideal for baking thick slices of bread or potatoes.

3. ROAST: With this function, you can cook poultry, minced meat, fish, vegetables, and sausages. Also great for browning the tops of grits, pots, and desserts.

4. BAKE: This function is used for baking your favorite cakes, muffins, and brownies.

5. ROAST: With this function, you can cook your favorite meat and poultry. You can also cook a whole chicken. Baking makes food tender and juicy inside.

6. HEAT: this function helps prevent the growth of bacteria. Keeps your oven temperature 160 ° C / 70 ° C.

7. PIZZA: This feature melts the cheese topping and browns on the top during pizza slices.

8. TEST: With this function, you can create the ideal environment to test the dough, slices of bread, slices of bread, and pizza.

9. AIRFRY: With these functions, you can make your food crisp and golden. This function is ideal for French fries.

10. HEAT: This function is ideal for reheating frozen food or food scraps without browning or drying the food.

11. COOKIES: This function is used for baking your favorite cookies and other baked goods.

12. BUY COOKING: This function is used for cooking your food for a long time at low temperatures.

13. Dehydration: This function is used to dry food without heating or to cook it. It is ideal for dehydrating your favorite fruits.

Advantages of the Smart Air Fryer Oven

The smart fryer oven comes with several benefits, some of which are as follows

• Healthy and fatty foods

The smart fryer oven works with transfer technology. Blow hot air into the cooking pan to cook food quickly and evenly on all sides. When frying your food in a smart fryer, you need a tablespoon or less than a tablespoon of oil. One bowl of fries requires only one tablespoon of oil and makes the fries crisp on the outside and tender on the inside. If you are amid the people who like fried food but are worried about extra calories, this kitchen appliance is for you.

• Offers 13-in-1 operation

The Breville smart air fryer oven offers 13 functions in one device. These functions are Toast, Bagel, Toast, Bake, Broil, Hot, Pizza, Proof, Air Fry, Reheat, Cookie, Slow Cook, and Dehydrate. These are all smart programs that offer flexible cooking.

• Safe to use

This is one of the safest frying methods compared to another traditional frying method. A narrow cooking method gives you a splatter-free cooking experience. Smart IQ technology makes the device safer, and there is no possibility of burning food. Smart IQ automatically detects and adjusts the temperature of the item according to the needs of the recipe.

• Easy to clean

The Breville smart fryer oven is made of reinforced stainless steel, and the inner body is coated with non-stick materials. All interior accessories are dishwasher safe. You can wash it in a dishwasher or also wash it with soapy water. The smart fryer cooks your food in much less oil. Less oil means less chaos.

CHAPTER 2:

Tips for Using Your Air fryer

One of the main problems facing families today is the excessive consumption of processed foods and fast foods, which are always high in fat, sugar and preservatives. One of the best ways to deal with this problem is by learning how to prepare healthy meals at home, but the problem is that cooking at home can be time consuming and requires a lot of equipment. This is where your Breville smart mini-oven comes in. Because it is very easy to use and clean, cooking at home is no longer a problem.

Breville Mini Smart Oven controls are easy to use that even a beginner can become a seasoned home cook in no time. After learning how it works, the whole family will want to join in the fun of cooking quickly, easy, and most importantly, healthy meals.

Preparing to Cook

- For the best finished result, pat off any excess moisture from the foods. This includes meat that has been soaked in a marinade and foods that have a high level of moisture, such as potatoes.
- You need very little oil when you cook with your air fryer, and some food will not require any oil at all. However, if you are not using any oil it is a good idea to use a little non-stick cooking spray applied directly to the food or the basket. This will help prevent your creation from sticking to the basket.
- When cutting an ingredient, try to keep the pieces uniform in size; this will ensure even cooking.
- Double check to make sure any fat drippings have been removed from the bottom of the air fryer after the previous use. Allowing fats and oils to accumulate will cause spattering and create smoke.
- When placing foods in the air fryer, remember to place them so there is plenty of room for air to circulate, even if it means cooking in batches. This will protect the quality of the finished dish and ensure even and proper cooking.
- Preheat the air fryer by setting it to the desired cooking temperature at least three to five minutes before you plan to start cooking.

During Cooking

- Note that recipes and cooking times are an approximation. Your pieces of meat, vegetables, etc. might be a different size or you may wish to alter the amounts of the ingredients. You might also prefer a different level of doneness. Adjust the cooking times up or down depending on the alterations you make, or to suit your individual taste. How closely packed the food is in the air fryer will also impact the amount of time needed for the dish to cook fully.

- Halfway through the cooking time, rotate your food. For smaller items such as fries, this means simply shaking the basket. Larger items should be flipped over.

Always Remember

The air fryer can add an exciting new element to your culinary repertoire. There is no reason you need to stick to traditional "fried" foods. This book will introduce you to additional dishes that can be created in your air fryer. This appliance is meant to be a healthy addition to your kitchen, and with some creativity and experimentation, you can add an incredible variety of fried, roasted, steamed, and baked dishes to your list of culinary creations.

CHAPTER 3:

Cleaning, Maintenance, And Positioning Of The Oven

Breville air fryer oven introduced a brand-new different air fryer kitchen appliance, which allows you to cook different food items in a healthier manner. This revolutionary air fryer is easy to clean due to its non-porous and non-stick interiors. Breville air fryer oven comes with different filters to purify the polluted air which is taken into the fryer. Hence you can cook food items without any risk of toxins or dust particles. The filters automatically clean the air before it going to the inside of the fryer.

Breville air fryer is easy to clean like a microwave or a toaster. You can simply clean the outer enclosure of the fryer by wiping it with a damp cloth which is usually equivalent to a wash. The filters you can clean by removing and cleaning it with soap and warm water.

Cleaning and maintenance of the parts

Breville air fryer oils are not supposed to be cleaned using a dishwasher for obvious reasons. The oils in your air fryer would mix with the dishwasher chemicals and then eventually it would be harmful. Hence we advise you to simply clean the outside and inner lid of the air fryer by removing the non-stick material in the lid and cleaning it with warm water and soap. You can simply remove the filter and clean it with warm water and soap also. If you want to clean the fryer in a simpler manner, you can use a wet towel or a wet paper towel to clean it. So, in total, the Breville air fryer oven is a home appliance you can use easily and maintain by following some basic instructions.

The positioning of the oven

You can easily place the Breville air fryer oven above your countertop. The fryer comes with a movable stand which allows you to change the position of your oven. You can place the fryer upwards to give a better view of the recipe book or even place it downwards if you want to maintain a lower profile. However, you can completely remove the feature of a stand as well. This freedom allows you to place it away from your countertop and fit it anywhere in your kitchen keeping your kitchen even more organized.

The safety features of the air fryer

Breville air fryer oven has been designed to keep your cooking safe and secure. The fryer has a digital timer which shows the exact time the food is being cooked. That way you can expect the food items to be ready at the scheduled time. It uses an electric heating system to cook the food, and hence it has a special door that you can close and lock. This feature of locking the door prevents the children or other people from accidentally opening it and hurting themselves.

The temperature of the air fryer

The temperature of food cooked in the Breville air fryer oven is measured in degrees Celsius, which seems to be a little bit weird for people who are more familiar with the Fahrenheit scale. This air fryer allows you to cook food items in a temperature range from 80 to 200 degrees Celsius. However, this fryer is not unable to cook food items with longer cooking times and if you want to cook food for a longer period of time, we advise you to cook it like a traditional oven.

The fryer is a great choice for weighted people and diet foods. It is not only easy to use but also very safe which is why it has been made to be truly environment friendly as well.

There are some more amazing features of this air fryer which are like it has a digital display for the user. This display allows you to have a real time understanding of how your food is being cooked as well. The display indicates the red zone and the recommended internal temperature. The recommended internal temperature is the last temperature range to cook any food item. This safety feature is perfect for chicken, meat, fish, etc. which if cooked beyond the temp range will make them lose a lot of their nutrients and tastes.

Breville have designed the Air Frier to be very user friendly. The instruction manual and recipe book that comes along with this air fryer are very simple and detailed also.

CHAPTER 4:

Breakfast

1. Breakfast Ham Omelet

Difficulty: Very Easy

Preparation Time: 10 minutes

Cooking Time: 10 minutes

Servings: 2

Ingredients:

- large eggs
- 100g ham, cut into small pieces
- ¼ cup milk
- ¾ cup mixed vegetables (white mushrooms, green onions, red pepper)
- ¼ cup mixed cheddar and mozzarella cheese
- 1 tsp. freshly chopped mixed herbs (cilantro and chives)
- Salt and freshly ground pepper to taste

Directions:

1. Mix the eggs and milk in a medium bowl then add in the remaining ingredients apart from the cheese and mixed herbs and beat well using a fork.
2. Pour the egg mix into an evenly greased pan then place it in the basket of your Breville smart air fryer toast oven.
3. Cook for roughly 10 minutes at 350°F or until done to desire.
4. Sprinkle the cheese and mixed herbs on the omelet halfway through cook time.
5. Gently loosen the omelet from the sides of the pan using a spatula.
6. Serve hot!

Nutrition:

Calories: 411 kcal/Cal

Carbs: 14 g

Fat: 39.3 g

Protein: 28 g

2. Breakfast Chicken Strips

Difficulty: Very Easy

Preparation Time: 5 minutes

Cooking Time: 12 minutes

Servings: 4

Ingredients:

- 1 teaspoon paprika
- 1 tablespoon cream
- 1 lb. chicken fillet
- ½ teaspoon salt
- ½ teaspoon black pepper

Directions:

1 Cut the chicken fillet into strips.

2 Sprinkle the chicken fillets with salt and pepper.

3 Preheat the air fryer to 365 degree Fahrenheit.

4 Place the butter in the air basket tray and add the chicken strips. Cook the chicken strips for 6-minutes.

5 Turn the chicken strips to the other side and cook them for an additional 5-minutes.
6 After strips are cooked, sprinkle them with cream and paprika, then transfer them to serving plates. Serve warm.

Nutrition:

Calories: 245,

Total Fat: 11.5g,

Carbs: 0.6g,

Protein: 33g

3. Citrus Blueberry Muffins

Difficulty: Very Easy

Preparation Time: 15 minutes

Cooking Time: 15 minutes

Servings: 3-4

Ingredients:

- 2 ½ cups cake flour
- ½ cup sugar
- ¼ cup light cooking oil such as avocado oil
- ½ cup heavy cream
- 1 cup fresh blueberries
- 2 eggs
- Zest and juice from 1 orange
- 1 tsp. pure vanilla extract
- 1 tsp. brown sugar for topping

Directions:

1 Start by combining the oil, heavy cream, eggs, orange juice and vanilla extract in a large bowl then set aside.
2 Separately combine the flour and sugar until evenly its mixed then pour little by little into the wet ingredients.
3 Combine until well blended but be careful not to over-mix.
4 Preheat your breville smart air fryer toast oven at 320°F
5 Fold the blueberries into the batter and split into cupcake holders, preferably, silicone cupcake holders as you won't have to grease them. Alternatively, you can use cupcake paper liners on any cupcake holders/ tray you could be having.
6 Dust the tops with the brown sugar and pop the muffins in the fryer.
7 Bake for about 12 minutes. Use a toothpick to check for readiness. When the muffins have evenly browned and an inserted toothpick comes out clean, they are ready.
8 Take out the muffins and let cool.
9 Enjoy!

Nutrition:

Calories: 289 kcal/Cal,

Carbs: 12.8 g

Fat: 32 g

Protein: 21.1 g

4. PB &J Donuts

Difficulty: Very Easy

Preparation Time: 15 minutes

Cooking Time: 12 minutes

Servings: 4

Ingredients:

- For the Donuts:
- 1 ¼ cups all-purpose flour
- ½ tsp. baking soda
- ½ tsp. baking powder

- 1/3 cup sugar
- ½ cup buttermilk
- 1 large egg
- 1 tsp. pure vanilla extract
- 3 tbsp. unsalted, melted and divided into 2+1
- ¾ tsp. salt
- For the Glaze:
- 2 tbsp. milk
- ½ cup powdered sugar
- 2 tbsp. smooth peanut butter
- Sea salt to taste
- For the Filling:
- ½ cup strawberry or blueberry jelly

Directions:

1 Mix all the dry ingredients for the donut in a large bowl.
2 Separately combine the egg, buttermilk, melted butter and vanilla extract.
3 Make a small well at the middle of the dry ingredients and pour in the egg mixture. Use a fork to join the ingredients then finish off with a spatula.
4 Place the dough on a floured surface and knead the dough. It will start out sticky but as you knead, it's going to come together.
5 Roll out the dough to make a ¾ inch thick circle. Use a cookie cutter, or the top part of a cup to cut the dough into rounds.
6 Place the donuts on a parchment paper and then into your Breville smart air fryer toast oven.
7 Cook for 12 minutes at 350°F.
8 Use a pastry bag to fill the donuts with jelly.
9 Combine the glaze ingredients and drizzle on top of the donuts.
10 Enjoy!

Nutrition:

Calories: 430 kcal/Cal

Carbs: 66.8 g

Fat: 14.6 g

Protein: 9.1 g

5. Breakfast Baked Apple

Difficulty: Very Easy

Preparation Time: 10 minutes

Cooking Time: 20 minutes

Servings: 2

Ingredients:

- 1 apple
- 2 tbsp. raisins
- 2 tbsp. walnuts, chopped
- ¼ tsp. nutmeg
- ¼ tsp. ground cinnamon
- 1 ½ tsp. margarine
- ¼ cup water

Directions:

1 Start by setting your Breville smart air fryer toast oven to 350°F.
2 Cut the apple in half and gently spoon out some of the flesh.
3 Place the apple halves on your Breville smart air fryer toast ovens frying pan.
4 Mix the raisins, walnuts, nutmeg, cinnamon and margarine in a bowl and divide equally between the apple halves.
5 Pour the water into the pan and cook for 20 minutes.
6 Enjoy!

Nutrition:

Calories: 161 kcal/Cal Carbs: 23.7 g Fat: 7.8 g

Protein: 2.5g

6. Sunny Side up Egg Tarts

Difficulty: Very Easy

Preparation Time: 15 minutes

Cooking Time: 20 minutes

Servings: 2

Ingredients:

- 4 eggs
- ¾ cup shredded Gruyere cheese (or preferred cheese)
- 1 sheet of puff pastry
- Minced chives for topping

Directions:

1 Start by flouring a clean surface then gently roll out your sheet of puff pastry and divide it into four equal squares.

2 If you have a small Breville smart air fryer toast oven, start with two squares but if it's big enough, go ahead and place the squares on the basket and cook for about 8-10 minutes or until they turn golden brown.

3 Whilst still in the basket, gently make an indentation at the center of each square and sprinkle 2-4 tablespoons of shredded cheese in the well then crack an egg on top.

4 Cook for 5-10 minutes or to desired doneness.

5 Remove from Breville smart air fryer toast oven, sprinkle with chives and you are ready to eat!

Nutrition:

Calories: 403 kcal/Cal

Carbs: 10.8 g

Fat: 29.4 g

Protein: 24.6 g

7. Healthy Spinach Scramble

Difficulty: Easy

Preparation Time: 8 minutes

Cooking Time: 30 minutes

Servings: 1

Ingredients:

- 3 egg whites
- 1 cup (packed) spinach
- 1 onion, chopped
- 2 tbsp. extra virgin olive oil
- ½ tsp. onion powder
- ½ tsp. garlic powder
- 1 tsp. turmeric powder
- Ground pepper to taste

Directions:

1 Preheat your Breville smart air fryer toast oven to 350°F.

2 Beat the egg whites and oil in a large bowl. Add in the fresh ingredients and mix until well combined then set the bowl aside.

3 Lightly grease your Breville smart air fryer toast oven's frying pan and transfer the egg mixture into the pan.

4 Cook in the fryer for about 10 minutes or until done to desire.

5 Serve hot.

Nutrition:

Calories: 285 kcal/Cal

Carbs: 12.3 g

Fat: 21.6 g

Protein: 13 g

8. Healthy Vegan Scramble

Difficulty: Easy

Preparation Time: 8 minutes

Cooking Time: 30 minutes

Servings: 3

Ingredients:

- 2 large potatoes, cut into cubes
- 1 tofu block, cut into cubes
- 1 broccoli, divided into florets
- 1 large onion, chopped
- 2 tbsp. dark soy sauce
- 2 tbsp. extra virgin olive oil, divided into 1+1
- ½ tsp. onion powder
- ½ tsp. garlic powder
- 1 tsp. turmeric powder
- Ground pepper to taste

Directions:

1 Start by marinating the tofu in 1 tablespoon of olive oil onion, garlic, turmeric and onion powders then set aside.

2 Drizzle the potatoes with the remaining tablespoon of olive oil and toss with pepper and cook in the Breville smart air fryer toast oven for 15 minutes at 400°F. Halfway through cook time, toss the potatoes to allow even cooking.

3 Toss the potatoes once more then mix in the marinated tofu, reserving the leftover liquid and cook for another 15 minutes at 370°F.

4 Toss the broccoli florets in the leftover marinade. If it's too little, drizzle with some soy sauce and toss to ensure all the florets are evenly covered.

5 When the potato-tofu mixture has 5 minutes of cooking time left, add in the broccoli.

6 Serve hot.

Nutrition:

Calories: 319 kcal/Cal

Carbs: 50.4 g

Fat: 10.9 g,

Protein: 8 g

9. Eggs in Zucchini Nest

Difficulty: Easy

Preparation Time: 5 minutes

Cooking Time: 7 minutes

Servings: 4

Ingredients:

- 4 teaspoons butter
- ½ teaspoon paprika
- ½ teaspoon black pepper
- ¼ teaspoon sea salt
- 4-ounces cheddar cheese, shredded
- 4 eggs
- 8-ounces zucchini, grated

Directions:

1 Grate the zucchini and place the butter in ramekins.

2 Add the grated zucchini in ramekins in the shape of nests. Sprinkle the zucchini nests with salt, pepper, and paprika.

3 Beat the eggs and pour over zucchini nests.

4 Top egg mixture with shredded cheddar cheese.

5 Preheat the air fryer basket and cook the dish for 7-minutes.

6 When the zucchini nests are cooked, chill them for 3-minutes and serve them in the ramekins.

Nutrition:

Calories: 221,

Total Fat: 17.7g,

Carbs: 2.9g,

Protein: 13.4g

10. Protein Egg Cups

Difficulty: Easy

Preparation Time: 10 minutes

Cooking Time: 9 minutes

Servings: 2

Ingredients:

- 3 eggs, lightly beaten
- 4 tomato slices
- 4 tsp cheddar cheese, shredded
- 2 bacon slices, cooked and crumbled
- Pepper
- Salt

Directions:

1 Spray silicone muffin molds with cooking spray.
2 Whisk the egg with pepper and salt in a bowl. Preheat the air fryer to 350 F.
3 Pour eggs into the silicone muffin molds. Divide cheese and bacon into molds.
4 Top each with tomato slice and place in the air fryer basket.
5 Cook for 9 minutes.
6 Serve and enjoy.

Nutrition:

Calories 67 Fat 4 g Carbohydrates 1 g

Sugar 0.7 g Protein 5.1 g Cholesterol 125 mg

11. Pumpkin Pancakes

Difficulty: Easy

Preparation Time: 15 minutes

Cooking Time: 12 minutes

Servings: 2

Ingredients:

- 1 square puff pastry
- 3 tablespoons pumpkin filling
- 1 small egg, beaten

Directions:

1 Roll out a square of puff pastry and layer it with pumpkin pie filling, leaving about ¼-inch space around the edges.
2 Cut it up into 8 equal sized square pieces and coat the edges with beaten egg.
3 Press "Power Button" of Air Fry Oven and turn the dial to select the "Air Fry" mode.
4 Press the Time button and again turn the dial to set the **Cooking Time:** to 12 minutes.
5 Push the Temp button and rotate the dial to set the temperature at 355 degrees F.
6 Press "Start/Pause" button to start.
7 When the unit beeps to show that it is preheated, open the lid.
8 Arrange the squares into a greased "Sheet Pan" and insert in the oven.
9 Serve warm.

Nutrition:

Calories 109 Total Fat 6.7 g

Saturated Fat 1.8 g Cholesterol 34 mg

Sodium 87 mg Total Carbs 9.8 g

Fiber 0.5 g Sugar 2.6 g

Protein 2.4 g

12. Shrimp Frittata

Difficulty: Easy

Preparation Time: 10 minutes

Cooking Time: 15 minutes

Servings: 2

Ingredients:

- 4 eggs
- ½ teaspoon basil, dried
- Cooking spray
- Salt and black pepper to the taste
- ½ cup rice, cooked
- ½ cup shrimp, cooked, peeled, deveined and chopped
- ½ cup baby spinach, chopped
- ½ cup Monterey jack cheese, grated

Directions:

1. Mix eggs with salt, pepper and basil and whisk.

1 Grease your air fryer's pan with cooking spray and add rice, shrimp and spinach.

2 Add eggs mix, sprinkle cheese all over and cook in your air fryer at 350 degrees F for 10 minutes.

3 Divide among plates and serve for breakfast.

4 Enjoy!

Nutrition:

Calories 162

Fat 6

Fiber 5

Carbs 8

Protein 4

13. Tuna Sandwiches

Difficulty: Easy

Preparation Time: 10 minutes

Cooking Time: 5 minutes

Servings: 2

Ingredients:

- 16 ounces canned tuna, drained
- ¼ cup mayonnaise
- 2 tablespoons mustard
- 1 tablespoons lemon juice
- 2 green onions, chopped
- 3 English muffins, halved
- 3 tablespoons butter
- provolone cheese

Directions:

1 In a bowl, mix tuna with mayo, lemon juice, mustard and green onions and stir. Grease muffin halves with the butter,

2 Place them in preheated air fryer and bake them at 350 degrees F for 4 minutes. Spread tuna mix on muffin halves,

3 top each with provolone cheese, return sandwiches to air fryer and cook them for 4 minutes,

4 Divide among plates and serve for breakfast right away.

5 Enjoy!

Nutrition:

Calories: 182

Fat: 4

Fiber: 7

Carbs: 8

Protein: 6

14. Cloud Eggs

Difficulty: Easy

Preparation Time: 8 minutes

Cooking Time: 4 minutes

Servings: 2

Ingredients:

- 1 teaspoon butter
- 2 eggs

Directions:

1 Separate the eggs and the egg yolks from the egg whites.
2 Then whisk the egg whites with the aid of the hand mixer until the white peaks are strong.
3 After that, spread the butter over the air fryer basket tray.
4 Heat up the air fryer to 300 F.
5 Get the egg white peaks medium clouds in the ready air fryer basket tray.
6 In the Air Fryer, position the basket tray and cook the cloud eggs for two minutes.
7 Take away the basket from the air Fryer after this, place the egg yolks in the middle of each egg cloud, and return the basket to the air fryer.
8 Cook the dish for an extra 2 minutes.
9 Then extract the cooked meal from the basket and serve.

Nutrition:

Calories 80,

Fat 6.3,

Fiber 0,

Carbs 0.3,

Protein 5.6

15. Chicken & Zucchini Omelet

Difficulty: Easy

Preparation Time: 15 minutes

Cooking Time: 35 minutes

Servings: 2

Ingredients:

- eggs
- ½ cup milk
- Salt and ground black pepper, as required
- 1 cup cooked chicken, chopped
- 1 cup Cheddar cheese, shredded
- ½ cup fresh chives, chopped
- ¾ cup zucchini, chopped

Directions:

1 Add the eggs, milk, salt and black pepper and beat well.
2 Add the remaining ingredients and stir to combine. Place the mixture into a greased baking pan. Press "Power Button" of Air Fry Oven and turn the dial to select the "Air Bake" mode. Press the Time button and again turn the dial to set the **Cooking Time:** to 35 minutes.
3 Now push the Temp button and rotate the dial to set the temperature at 315 degrees F. Press "Start/Pause" button to start. When the unit beeps to show that it is preheated, open the lid.
4 Arrange pan over the "Wire Rack" and insert in the oven. Cut into equal-sized wedges and serve hot.

Nutrition:

Calories: 209 Total Fat: 13.3 g Saturated Fat: 6.3 g

Cholesterol: 258 mg Sodium: 252 mg

Total Carbs: 2.3 g Fiber: 0.3 g Sugar: 1.8 g

Protein: 9.8 g

16. Zucchini Fritters

Difficulty: Medium

Preparation Time: 15 minutes

Cooking Time: 7 minutes

Servings: 2

Ingredients:

- 10½ oz. zucchini, grated and squeezed
- oz. Halloumi cheese
- ¼ cup all-purpose flour
- 2 eggs
- 1 teaspoon fresh dill, minced
- Salt and ground black pepper, as required

Directions:

1 In a large bowl and mix together all the ingredients. Make a small-sized fritter from the mixture.

2 Press "Power Button" of Air Fry Oven and turn the dial to select the "Air Fry" mode. Press the Time button and again turn the dial to set the **Cooking Time:** to 7 minutes.

3 Now push the Temp button and rotate the dial to set the temperature at 355 degrees F. Press "Start/Pause" button to start.

4 When the unit beeps to show that it is preheated, open the lid. Arrange fritters into grease "Sheet Pan" and insert in the oven.

5 Serve warm.

Nutrition:

Calories: 253

Total Fat: 17.2 g

Saturated Fat: 11 g

Cholesterol: 121 mg

Sodium: 333 mg

Total Carbs: 10 g

Fiber: 1.1 g

Sugar: 2.7 g

Protein: 15.2 g

17. Onion Omelet

Difficulty: Medium

Preparation Time: 10 minutes

Cooking Time: 15 minutes

Servings: 2

Ingredients:

- eggs
- ¼ teaspoon low-sodium soy sauce
- Ground black pepper, as required
- 1 teaspoon butter
- 1 medium yellow onion, sliced
- ¼ cup Cheddar cheese, grated

Directions:

1 In a skillet, melt the butter over medium heat and cook the onion and cook for about 8-10 minutes.

2 Remove from the heat and set aside to cool slightly.

3 Meanwhile, in a bowl, add the eggs, soy sauce and black pepper and beat well.

4 Add the cooked onion and gently, stir to combine. Place the zucchini mixture into a small baking pan.

5 Press "Power Button" of Air Fry Oven and turn the dial to select the "Air Fry" mode.

6 Press the Time button and again turn the dial to set the cooking time to 5 minutes.

7 Now push the Temp button and rotate the dial to set the temperature at 255

degrees F. Press "Start/Pause" button to start.

8 When the unit beeps to show that it is preheated,

9 Open the lid. Arrange pan over the "Wire Rack" and insert in the oven.

10 Cut the omelet into 2 portions and serve hot.

Nutrition:

Calories: 222

Total Fat: 15.4 g

Saturated Fat: 6.9 g

Cholesterol: 347 mg

Sodium: 264 mg

Total Carbs: 6.1 g

Fiber: 1.2 g Sugar: 3.1 g Protein: 15.3 g

18. Egg Cups with Bacon

Difficulty: Medium

Preparation Time: 10 minutes

Cooking Time: 15 minutes

Servings: 4

Ingredients:

- ½ teaspoon paprika
- 1 tablespoon butter
- ¼ teaspoon salt
- ½ teaspoon dried dill
- eggs
- oz. bacon

Directions:

1 In the blender pot, beat the eggs. Paprika, salt, and dried dill are then added. Using the hand blender, carefully mix the egg mixture.

2 Then pour the butter over four ramekins.

3 Cut the bacon and put it in cup shape in ready-made ramekins.

4 Dress the egg mix with bacon in the middle of each ramekin.

5 Put Air fryer at 360 F.

6 Put the ramekins in the Air fryer and cover it.

7 Cook for 15 minutes.

8 When the time is finished, the mixture of eggs and bacon should be delicious.

9 Take out the egg cups and serve.

Nutrition:

Calories 319, Fat 25.1, Fiber 0.1,

Carbs 1.2, Protein 21.4

19. Almond Crust Chicken

Difficulty: Medium

Preparation Time: 10 minutes

Cooking Time: 25 minutes

Servings: 2

Ingredients:

- 2 chicken breasts, skinless and boneless
- 1 tbsp. Dijon mustard
- 2 tbsp. mayonnaise
- ¼ cup almonds
- Pepper
- Salt

Directions:

1 Add almond into the food processor and process until finely ground. Transfer almonds on a plate and set aside.

2 Mix together mustard and mayonnaise and spread over chicken.

3 Coat chicken with almond and place into the air fryer basket and cook at 350 F for 25 minutes
4 . Serve and enjoy.

Nutrition:

Calories 409 Fat 22 g

Carbohydrates 6 g Sugar 1.5 g

Protein 45 g

Cholesterol 134 mg

20. Potatoes with Bacon

Difficulty: Medium

Preparation Time: 10 minutes

Cooking Time: 20 minutes

Servings: 2

Ingredients:

- potatoes, peeled and cut into medium cubes
- garlic cloves, minced
- bacon slices, chopped
- 2 rosemary springs, chopped
- 1 tablespoon olive oil
- Salt and black pepper to the taste
- 2 eggs, whisked

Directions:

1 In your air fryer's pan, mix oil with potatoes, garlic, bacon, rosemary, salt, pepper and eggs and whisk.
2 Cook potatoes at 400 degrees F for 20 minutes,
3 Divide everything on plates and serve for breakfast.
4 Enjoy!

Nutrition:

Calories: 211

Fat: 3

Fiber: 5

Carbs: 8

Protein: 5

21. Zucchini Squash Mix

Difficulty: Medium

Preparation Time: 10 minutes

Cooking Time: 35 minutes

Servings: 2

Ingredients:

- 1 lb. zucchini, sliced
- 1 tbsp. parsley, chopped
- 1 yellow squash, halved, deseeded, and chopped
- 1 tbsp. olive oil
- Pepper
- Salt

Directions:

1 Place all ingredients into the large bowl and mix well.
2 Transfer bowl mixture into the air fryer basket and cook at 400 F for 35 minutes.
3 Serve and enjoy.

Nutrition:

Calories: 49

Fat: 3 g

Carbohydrates: 4 g

Sugar: 2 g

Protein: 1.5 g

Cholesterol: 0 mg

22. Special Corn Flakes Casserole

Difficulty: Hard

Preparation Time: 10 minutes

Cooking Time: 18 Minutes

Servings: 5

Ingredients:

- 1/3 cup milk
- tbsp. cream cheese; whipped
- 1/4 tsp. nutmeg; ground
- 1/4 cup blueberries
- 1 ½ cups corn flakes; crumbled
- 3 tsp. sugar
- 2 eggs; whisked
- bread slices

Directions:

1 In a bowl; mix eggs with sugar, nutmeg and milk and whisk well.

2 In another bowl; mix cream cheese with blueberries and whisk well.

3 Put corn flakes in a third bowl.

4 Spread blueberry mix on each bread slice; then dip in eggs mix and dredge in corn flakes at the end.

5 Place bread in your air fryer's basket; heat up at 400 °F and bake for 8 minutes.

6 Divide among plates and serve for breakfast.

Nutrition:

Calories: 300;

Fat: 5;

Fiber: 7;

Carbs: 16;

Protein: 4

23. Protein Rich Egg White Omelet

Difficulty: Hard

Preparation Time: 10 minutes

Cooking Time: 25 Minutes

Servings: 4

Ingredients:

- 1 cup egg whites
- 1/4 cup mushrooms; chopped
- 2 tbsp. chives; chopped
- 1/4 cup tomato; chopped
- 2 tbsp. skim milk
- Salt and black pepper to the taste

Directions:

1 In a bowl; mix egg whites with tomato, milk, mushrooms, chives, salt and pepper;

2 Whisk well and pour into your air fryer's pan. Cook at 320 °F, for 15 minutes;

3 Cool omelet down, slice, divide among plates and serve.

Nutrition:

Calories: 100; Fat: 3; Fiber: 6;

Carbs: 7; Carbs: 4

24. Shrimp Sandwiche

Difficulty: Hard

Preparation Time: 10 minutes

Cooking Time: 15 Minutes

Servings: 4

Ingredients:

- 1 ¼ cups cheddar; shredded
- 2 tbsp. green onions; chopped.

- whole wheat bread slices
- oz. canned tiny shrimp; drained
- tbsp. mayonnaise
- 2 tbsp. butter; soft

Directions:

1 In a bowl; mix shrimp with cheese, green onion and mayo and stir well.
2 Spread this on part of the bread slices; top with the other bread slices, cut into halves diagonally and spread butter on top.
3 Place sandwiches in your air fryer and cook at 350 °F, for 5 minutes. Divide shrimp sandwiches on plates and serve them for breakfast.

Nutrition:

Calories: 162; Fat: 3; Fiber: 7;

Carbs: 12; Protein: 4

25. Breakfast Soufflé

Difficulty: Hard

Preparation Time: 10 minutes

Cooking Time: 18 Minutes

Servings: 4

Ingredients:

- eggs; whisked
- tbsp. heavy cream
- 2 tbsp. parsley; chopped.
- 2 tbsp. chives; chopped.
- A pinch of red chili pepper; crushed
- Salt and black pepper to the taste

Directions:

1. Mix the eggs with salt, pepper, heavy cream, red pepper, parsley, and chives. Mix well and divide into 4 soufflé plates.
2. Place the dishes in your deep fryer and cook the soufflé at 350 ° F for 8 minutes. Serve hot.

Nutrition: Calories:

300; Fat: 7; Fiber: 9; Carbs: 15; Protein: 6

26. Fried Tomato Quiche

Difficulty: Hard

Preparation Time: 10 minutes

Cooking Time: 40 Minutes

Servings: 1

Ingredients:

- 1 tbsp. yellow onion; chopped.
- 1/2 cup gouda cheese; shredded
- 1/4 cup tomatoes; chopped.
- 2 eggs
- 1/4 cup milk
- Salt and black pepper to the taste
- Cooking spray

Directions:

1 Grease a ramekin with cooking spray.
2 Crack eggs, add onion, milk, cheese, tomatoes, salt and pepper and stir. Add this in your air fryer's pan and cook at 340 °F, for 30 minutes.

Nutrition:

Calories: 241;

Fat: 6;

Fiber: 8;

Carbs: 14;

Protein: 6

27. Breakfast Spanish Omelet

Difficulty: Hard

Preparation Time: 10 minutes

Cooking Time: 20 Minutes

Servings: 4

Ingredients:

- eggs
- 1/2 chorizo; chopped
- 1 tbsp. parsley; chopped.
- 1 tbsp. feta cheese; crumbled
- 1 potato; peeled and cubed
- 1/2 cup corn
- 1 tbsp. olive oil
- Salt and black pepper to the taste

Directions:

1 Heat up your air fryer at 350 °F and add oil.

2 Add chorizo and potatoes; stir and brown them for a few seconds.

3 In a bowl; mix eggs with corn, parsley, cheese, salt and pepper and whisk.

4 Pour this over chorizo and potatoes; spread and cook for 5 minutes. Divide omelet on plates and serve for breakfast.

Nutrition:

Calories: 300;

Fat: 6;

Fiber: 9;

Carbs: 12;

Protein: 6

28. Scrambled Pancake Hash

Difficulty: Hard

Preparation Time: 5 minutes

Cooking Time: 9 minutes

Servings: 7

Ingredients:

- 1 egg
- ¼ cup heavy cream
- tablespoons butter
- 1 cup coconut flour
- 1 teaspoon ground ginger
- 1 teaspoon salt
- 1 tablespoon apple cider vinegar
- 1 teaspoon baking soda

Directions:

1. Combine the salt, baking soda, ground ginger and flour in a mixing bowl. In a separate bowl crack, the egg into it.
2. Add butter and heavy cream.
3. Mix well using a hand mixer. Combine the liquid and dry mixtures and stir until smooth.
4. Preheat your air fryer to 400 degree Fahrenheit. Pour the pancake mixture into the air fryer basket tray.
5. Cook the pancake hash for 4-minutes.
6. After this, scramble the pancake hash well and continue to cook for another 5-minutes more.
7. When dish is cooked, transfer it to serving plates, and serve hot!

Nutrition:

Calories: 178, Total Fat: 13.3g,

Carbs: 10.7g, Protein: 4.4g

29. Onion Frittata

Difficulty: Hard

Preparation Time: 20 minutes

Cooking Time: 30 Minutes

Servings: 6

Ingredients:

- eggs; whisked
- 1 tbsp. olive oil
- 1 lb. small potatoes; chopped
- 1 oz. cheddar cheese; grated
- 1/2 cup sour cream
- yellow onions; chopped
- Salt and black pepper to the taste

Directions:

1. In a large bowl; mix eggs with potatoes, onions, salt, pepper, cheese and sour cream and whisk well.
2. Grease your air fryer's pan with the oil, add eggs mix; place in air fryer and cook for 20 minutes at 320 degrees F. Slice frittata, divide among plates and serve for breakfast.

Nutrition:

Calories: 231; Fat: 5; Fiber: 7;

Carbs: 8; Protein: 4

30. Pea Tortilla

Difficulty: Very Hard

Preparation Time: 10 minutes

Cooking Time: 17 Minutes

Servings: 8

Ingredients:

- 1/2 lb. baby peas
- 1 ½ cup yogurt
- eggs
- 1/2 cup mint; chopped.
- tbsp. butter
- Salt and black pepper to the taste

Directions:

1. Heat up a pan that fits your air fryer with the butter over medium heat, add peas; mix and cook for a couple of minutes.
2. Meanwhile; in a bowl, mix half of the yogurt with salt, pepper, eggs and mint and whisk well.
3. Pour this over the peas, toss, introduce in your air fryer and cook at 350 °F, for 7 minutes. Spread the rest of the yogurt over your tortilla; slice and serve.

Nutrition:

Calories: 192; Fat: 5;

Fiber: 4; Carbs: 8; Protein: 7

31. Mushroom Quiches

Difficulty: Very Hard

Preparation Time: 10 minutes

Cooking Time: 20 Minutes

Servings: 4

Ingredients:

- Button mushrooms; chopped.
- tbsp. ham; chopped
- eggs
- 1 tbsp. flour
- 1 tbsp. butter; soft
- 9-inch pie dough
- 1/2 tsp. thyme; dried
- 1/4 cup Swiss cheese; grated

- 1 small yellow onion; chopped.
- 1/3 cup heavy cream
- A pinch of nutmeg; ground
- Salt and black pepper to the taste

Directions:

1 Dust a working surface with the flour and roll the pie dough.
2 Press in on the bottom of the pie pan your air fryer has.
3 In a bowl; mix butter with mushrooms, ham, onion, eggs, heavy cream, salt, pepper, thyme and nutmeg and whisk well.
4 Add this over pie crust, spread, sprinkle Swiss cheese all over and place pie pan in your air fryer.
5 Cook your quiche at 400 °F, for 10 minutes. Slice and serve for breakfast.

Nutrition:

Calories: 212;

Fat: 4;

Fiber: 6;

Carbs: 7;

Protein: 7

32. Walnuts Pear Oatmeal

Difficulty: Very Hard

Preparation Time: 10 minutes

Cooking Time: 17 Minutes

Servings: 4

Ingredients:

- 1 tbsp. butter; soft
- 1/4 cups brown sugar
- 1 cup water
- 1/2 cup raisins
- 1/2 tsp. cinnamon powder
- 1 cup rolled oats
- 1/2 cup walnuts; chopped.
- 2 cups pear; peeled and chopped.

Directions:

1 Mix milk with sugar, butter, oats, cinnamon, raisins, pears and walnuts; stir,
2 Introduce in your fryer and cook at 360 °F, for 12 minutes.
3 Divide into bowls and serve.

Nutrition:

Calories: 230;

Fat: 6;

Fiber: 11;

Carbs: 20;

Protein: 5

33. Breakfast Raspberry Rolls

Difficulty: Very Hard

Preparation Time: 10 minutes

Cooking Time: 50 Minutes

Servings: 6

Ingredients:

- 1 cup milk
- 1/4 cup sugar
- 1 egg
- tbsp. butter
- ¼ cups flour
- tsp. yeast
- For the filling:
- oz. cream cheese; soft
- oz. raspberries
- 1 tsp. vanilla extract

- tbsp. sugar
- 1 tbsp. cornstarch
- Zest from 1 lemon; grated

Directions:

Mix flour with sugar and yeast and stir.

1 Add milk and egg, stir until you obtain a dough, leave it aside to rise for 30 minutes; transfer dough to a working surface and roll well.

2 Mix cream cheese with sugar, vanilla and lemon zest; stir well and spread over dough.

3 In another bowl; mix raspberries with cornstarch, stir and spread over cream cheese mix.

4 Roll your dough, cut into medium pieces, place them in your air fryer; spray them with cooking spray and cook them at 350 °F, for 30 minutes. Serve your rolls for breakfast.

Nutrition:

Calories: 261; Fat: 5; Fiber: 8;

Carbs: 9; Protein: 6

34. Bread Pudding

Difficulty: Very Hard

Preparation Time: 10 minutes

Cooking Time: 32 Minutes

Servings: 4

Ingredients:

- 1/2 lb. white bread; cubed
- 3/4 cup milk
- 3/4 cup water
- tsp. cinnamon powder
- 1 cup flour
- 3/5 cup brown sugar
- tsp. cornstarch
- 1/2 cup apple; peeled; cored and roughly chopped.
- 1 tbsp. honey
- 1 tsp. vanilla extract
- oz. soft butter

Directions:

1 In a bowl; mix bread with apple, milk with water, honey, cinnamon, vanilla and cornstarch and whisk well.

2 Mix flour with sugar and butter and stir until you obtain a crumbled mixture.

3 Press half of the crumble mix on the bottom of your air fryer; add bread and apple mix, add the rest of the crumble and cook everything at 350 °F, for 22 minutes. Divide bread pudding on plates and serve.

Nutrition:

Calories: 261; Fat: 7; Fiber: 7;

Carbs: 8; Protein: 5

35. Cream Cheese Oats

Difficulty: Very Hard

Preparation Time: 10 minutes

Cooking Time: 35 Minutes

Servings: 4

Ingredients:

- 1 cup steel oats
- cups milk
- 1 tbsp. butter
- tbsp. white sugar
- oz. cream cheese; soft
- 3/4 cup raisins

- 1 tsp. cinnamon powder
- 1/4 cup brown sugar

Directions:

1 Heat up a pan that fits your air fryer with the butter over medium heat, add oats; stir and toast them for 3 minutes.
2 Add milk and raisins; stir, introduce in your air fryer and cook at 350 °F, for 20 minutes.
3 Meanwhile; in a bowl, mix cinnamon with brown sugar and stir.
4 In a second bowl; mix white sugar with cream cheese and whisk. Divide oats into bowls and top each with cinnamon and cream cheese.

Nutrition:

Calories: 152;

Fat: 6;

Fiber: 6;

Carbs: 25;

Protein: 7

36. Bread Rolls

Difficulty: Very Hard

Preparation Time: 10 minutes

Cooking Time: 22 Minutes

Servings: 4

Ingredients:

- potatoes; boiled; peeled and mashed
- 1/2 tsp. turmeric powder
- curry leaf springs
- 1/2 tsp. mustard seeds
- bread slices; white parts only
- 1 coriander bunch; chopped.
- green chilies; chopped
- Small yellow onions; chopped.
- 2 tbsp. olive oil
- Salt and black pepper to the taste

Directions:

1 Heat up a pan with 1 tsp. oil; add mustard seeds, onions, curry leaves and turmeric, stir and cook for a few seconds.
2 Add mashed potatoes, salt, pepper, coriander and chilies, stir well; take off heat and cool it down.
3 Divide potatoes mix into 8 parts and shape ovals using your wet hands.
4 Wet bread slices with water; press in order to drain excess water and keep one slice in your palm.
5 Add a potato oval over bread slice and wrap it around it.
6 Do the same with the rest of the potato mix and bread.
7 Heat up your air fryer at 400 degrees F; add the rest of the oil, add bread rolls; cook them for 12 minutes. Divide bread rolls on plates and serve for breakfast.

Nutrition:

Calories: 261;

Fat: 6;

Fiber: 9;

Carbs: 12;

Protein: 7

CHAPTER 5:

Lunch

37. Rolled Salmon Sandwich

Difficulty: Very Easy

Preparation Time: 5 minutes

Cooking time: 5 minutes

Servings: 1

Ingredients:

- 1 piece of flatbread
- 1 salmon filet
- Pinch of salt
- 1 tablespoon green onion, chopped
- 1/4 teaspoon dried sumac
- 1/2 teaspoon thyme
- 1/2 teaspoon sesame seeds
- 1/4 English cucumber
- 1 tablespoon yogurt

Directions:

1. Start by peeling and chopping the cucumber. Cut the salmon at a 45-degree angle into 4 slices and lay them flat on the flatbread.
2. Sprinkle salmon with salt to taste. Sprinkle onions, thyme, sumac, and sesame seeds evenly over the salmon.
3. Broil the salmon for at least 3 minutes, but longer if you want a more well-done fish.
4. While you broil your salmon, mix the yogurt and cucumber. Remove your flatbread from the toaster oven, put it on a plate, and spoon the yogurt mix over the salmon.
5. Fold the flatbread sides in and roll it up for a gourmet lunch that you can take on the go.

Nutrition:

Calories: 347,

Sodium: 397 mg,

Dietary Fiber: 1.6 g,

Total Fat: 12.4 g,

Total Carbs: 20.6 g,

Protein: 38.9 g.

38. Balsamic Roasted Chicken

Difficulty: Very Easy

Preparation Time: 10 minutes

Cooking time: 1 hour

Servings: 4

Ingredients:

- 1/2 cup balsamic vinegar
- 1/4 cup Dijon mustard
- 1/3 cup olive oil
- Juice and zest from 1 lemon

- minced garlic cloves
- 1 teaspoon salt
- 1 teaspoon pepper
- bone-in, skin-on chicken thighs
- bone-in, skin-on chicken drumsticks
- 1 tablespoon chopped parsley

Directions:

1. Mix vinegar, lemon juice, mustard, olive oil, garlic, salt, and pepper in a bowl and then pour it into a saucepan.
2. Roll chicken pieces in the pan, then cover and marinate for at least 2 hours, but up to 24 hours.
3. Preheat the oven to 400°F and place the chicken on a fresh baking sheet, reserving the marinade later.
4. Roast the chicken for 50 minutes.
5. Take the chicken and cover it with foil to keep it warm. Place the marinade in the toaster oven for about 5 minutes until it simmers down and begins to thicken.
6. Pour marinade over chicken and sprinkle with parsley and lemon zest.

Nutrition:

Calories: 1537,

Sodium: 1383 mg,

Dietary

Fiber: 0.8 g,

Total Fat: 70.5 g,

Total Carbs: 2.4 g,

Protein: 210.4 g.

39. Chicken Capers Sandwich

Difficulty: Very Easy

Preparation Time: 3 minutes

Cooking time: 3 minutes

Servings: 2

Ingredients:

- leftover chicken breasts or pre-cooked breaded chicken
- 1 large ripe tomato
- ounces' mozzarella cheese slices
- slices of whole-grain bread
- 1/4 cup olive oil
- 1/3 cup fresh basil leaves
- Salt and pepper to taste

Directions:

1 Start by slicing tomatoes into thin slices.

2 Layer tomatoes, then cheese over two slices of bread and place on a greased baking sheet.

3 Grill for about 3 minutes

4 Heat chicken while the cheese melts.

5 Remove from oven, sprinkle with basil, and add chicken.

6 Sprinkle with oil and add salt and pepper. Top with other slices of bread and serve.

Nutrition:

Calories: 808, Sodium: 847 mg,

Dietary Fiber: 5.2 g, Total Fat: 43.6 g,

Total Carbs: 30.7 g, Protein: 78.4 g.

40. Easy Prosciutto Grilled Cheese

Difficulty: Very Easy

Preparation Time: 5 minutes

Cooking time: 5 minutes

Servings: 1

Ingredients:

- slices muenster cheese
- slices white bread
- Four thinly-shaved pieces of prosciutto
- 1 tablespoon sweet and spicy pickles

Directions:

1 Set toaster oven to the Toast setting.

2 Put one slice of cheese on each piece of bread. Put prosciutto on one slice and pickles on the other.

3 Take it to a baking sheet and toast for 4 minutes or until the cheese is melted. Combine the sides, cut, and serve.

Nutrition:

Calories: 460, Sodium: 2180 mg,

Dietary Fiber: 0 g, Total Fat: 25.2 g,

Total Carbs: 11.9 g, Protein: 44.2 g.

41. Herb-Roasted Chicken Tenders

Difficulty: Very Easy

Preparation Time: 5 minutes

Cooking time: 10 minutes

Servings: 2

Ingredients:

- ounces' chicken tenders
- 1 tablespoon olive oil
- 1/2 teaspoon Herbes de Provence
- tablespoons Dijon mustard
- 1 tablespoon honey
- Salt and pepper

Directions:

1 Start by preheating the toaster oven to 450°F.

2 Brush the bottom of the pan with 1/2 tablespoon olive oil.

3 Spice the chicken with herbs, salt, and pepper.

4 Place the chicken in a single flat layer in the pan and drizzle the remaining olive oil over it.

5 Bake for about 10 minutes.

6 While the chicken is baking, mix the mustard and honey for a tasty condiment.

Nutrition:

Calories: 297, Sodium: 268 mg,

Dietary Fiber: 0.8 g, Total Fat: 15.5 g,

Total Carbs: 9.6 g, Protein: 29.8 g.

42. Moroccan Pork Kebabs

Difficulty: Very Easy

Preparation Time: 40 minutes

Cooking time: 45 minutes

Servings: 4

Ingredients:

- 1/4 cup orange juice

- 1 tablespoon tomato paste
- 1 clove chopped garlic
- 1 tablespoon ground cumin
- 1/8 teaspoon ground cinnamon
- tablespoons olive oil
- 1-1/2 teaspoons salt
- 3/4 teaspoon black pepper
- 1-1/2 pounds' boneless pork loin
- 1 small eggplant
- 1 small red onion
- Pita bread (optional)
- 1/2 small cucumber
- tablespoons chopped fresh mint
- Wooden skewers

Directions:

1. Begin by placing wooden skewers in water to soak.
2. Cut pork loin and eggplant into 1- to 1-1/2-inch chunks.
3. Preheat toaster oven to 425°F.
4. Cut cucumber and onions into pieces and chop the mint.
5. Combine the orange juice, tomato paste, garlic, cumin, and cinnamon, 2 tablespoons of oil, 1 teaspoon of salt, and 1/2 teaspoon of pepper.
6. Add the pork to this mixture and refrigerate for at least 30 minutes, but up to 8 hours.
7. Mix vegetables, remaining oil, and salt and pepper.
8. Skewer the vegetables and bake for 20 minutes.
9. Add the pork to the skewers and bake for an additional 25 minutes.
10. Remove ingredients from skewers and sprinkle with mint; serve with flatbread if using.

Nutrition:

Calories: 465,

Sodium: 1061 mg,

Dietary Fiber: 5.6 g,

Total Fat: 20.8 g,

Total Carbs: 21.9 g,

Protein: 48.2 g.

43. Pecan Crunch Catfish and Asparagus

Difficulty: Very Easy

Preparation Time: 5 minutes

Cooking time: 12 minutes

Servings: 4

Ingredients:

- 1 cup whole-wheat panko breadcrumbs
- 1/4 cup chopped pecans
- teaspoons chopped fresh thyme
- 1-1/2 tablespoons extra-virgin olive oil, plus more for the pan
- Salt and pepper to taste
- 1-1/4 pounds' asparagus
- 1 tablespoon honey
- (5- to 6-ounce each) catfish filets

Directions:

1 Start by preheating the toaster oven to 425°F.

2 Combine breadcrumbs, pecans, 2 teaspoons thyme, 1 tablespoon oil, salt, pepper, and 2 tablespoons water.

3 In another bowl, combine asparagus, the rest of the thyme, honey, salt, and pepper.

4 Spread the asparagus in a flat layer on a baking sheet. Sprinkle a quarter of the breadcrumb mixture over the asparagus.

5 Lay the catfish over the asparagus and press the rest of the breadcrumb mixture into each piece—roast for 12 minutes.

Nutrition:

Calories: 531,

Sodium: 291 mg,

Dietary Fiber: 6.1 g,

Total Fat: 30.4 g,

Total Carbs: 31.9 g,

Protein: 34.8 g.

44. Parmesan-Crusted Pork Loi

Difficulty: Very Easy

Preparation Time: 10 minutes

Cooking time: 20 minutes

Servings: 4

Ingredients:

- 1-pound pork loin
- 1 teaspoon salt
- 1/2 tablespoon garlic powder
- 1/2 tablespoon onion powder
- tablespoons parmesan cheese
- 1 tablespoon olive oil

Directions:

1 Start by preheating the toaster oven to 475°F.

2 Put the pan in the oven and let it heat while the oven preheats.

3 Mix all ingredients in a shallow dish and roll the pork loin until it is fully coated.

4 Remove pan and sear the pork in the pan on each side.

5 Once seared, bake pork in the pan for 20 minutes.

Nutrition:

Calories: 334, Sodium: 718 mg,

Dietary Fiber: 0 g, Total Fat: 20.8 g,

Total Carbs: 1.7 g, Protein: 33.5 g.

45. Persimmon Toast with Sour Cream & Cinnamon

Difficulty: Very Easy

Preparation Time: 5 minutes

Cooking time: 5 minutes

Servings: 1

Ingredients:

- 1 slice of wheat bread
- 1/2 persimmon
- Sour cream to taste

- Sugar to taste
- Cinnamon to taste

Directions:

1 Apply a thin layer of sour cream across the bread.

2 Slice the persimmon into 1/4 inch pieces and lay them across the bread.

3 Sprinkle cinnamon and sugar over persimmon.

4 Toast in the toaster oven until bread and persimmon begin to brown.

Nutrition:

Calories: 89,

Sodium: 133 mg,

Dietary Fiber: 2.0 g,

Total Fat: 1.1 g,

Total Carbs: 16.5 g,

Protein: 3.8 g.

46. Roasted Beet Salad with Oranges & Beet Greens

Difficulty: Very Easy

Preparation Time: 7 minutes

Cooking time: 10 minutes

Servings: 6

Ingredients:

- medium beets with beet greens attached
- large oranges
- 1 small sweet onion, cut into wedges
- 1/3 cup red wine vinegar
- 1/4 cup extra-virgin olive oil
- garlic cloves, minced
- 1/2 teaspoon grated orange peel

Directions:

1 Start by preheating the toaster oven to 400°F.

2 Trim leaves from beets and chop, then set aside.

3 Pierce beets with a fork and place in a roasting pan.

4 Roast beets for 1-1/2 hours.

5 Allow beets to cool, peel then cut into 8 wedges and put into a bowl.

6 Place beet greens in a saucepan and cover with just enough water to cover. Heat until water boils, then immediately remove from heat.

7 Drain greens and press to remove liquid from greens, then add to beet bowl.

8 Remove peel and pith from orange and segment, adding each part to the bowl.

9 Add onion to beet mixture. In a separate bowl, mix vinegar, oil, garlic, and orange peel.

10 Combine both bowls and toss, sprinkle with salt and pepper.

11 Let stand for an hour before serving.

Nutrition:

Calories: 214, Sodium: 183 mg,

Dietary Fiber: 6.5 g,

Total Fat: 8.9 g,

Total Carbs: 32.4 g,

Protein: 4.7 g.

47. Roasted Grape and Goat Cheese Crostinis

Difficulty: Very Easy

Preparation Time: 30 minutes

Cooking time: 5 minutes

Servings: 10

Ingredients:

- 1 pound seedless red grapes
- 1 teaspoon chopped rosemary
- tablespoons olive oil
- 1 rustic French baguette
- 1 cup sliced shallots
- tablespoons unsalted butter
- ounces' goat cheese
- 1 tablespoon honey

Directions:

1 Start by preheating the toaster oven to 400°F.

2 Toss grapes, rosemary, and 1 tablespoon of olive oil in a large bowl.

3 Take it to a roasting pan and roast for 20 minutes.

4 Remove the pan from the oven and set aside to cool.

5 Slice the baguette into 1/2-inch-thick pieces.

6 Rub each slice with olive oil and place on a baking sheet.

7 Cook for 8 minutes, then remove from oven and set aside.

8 In a medium skillet, add butter and one tablespoon of olive oil.

9 Add shallots and sauté for about 10 minutes.

10 Mix goat cheese and honey in a medium bowl, then add the shallot pan and mix thoroughly.

11 Spread shallot mixture onto a baguette, top with grapes, and serve.

Nutrition:

Calories: 238, Sodium: 139 mg,

Dietary Fiber: 0.6 g, Total Fat: 16.3 g,

Total Carbs: 16.4 g, Protein: 8.4 g.

48. Roasted Mini Peppers

Difficulty: Very Easy

Preparation Time: 2 minutes

Cooking time: 10 minutes

Servings: 6

Ingredients:

- 1 bag mini bell peppers
- Cooking spray
- Salt and pepper to taste

Directions:

1 Start by preheating the toaster oven to 400°F.

2 Wash and dry the peppers, then place flat on a baking sheet.

3 Spray peppers with cooking spray and sprinkle with salt and pepper.

4 Roast for 15 minutes.

Nutrition:

Calories: 19, Sodium: 2 mg, Dietary Fiber: 1.3 g,

Total Fat: 0.3 g, Total Carbs: 3.6 g, Protein: 0.6 g.

49. Skinny Black Bean Flautas

Difficulty: Easy

Preparation Time: 10 minutes

Cooking time: 25 minutes

Servings: 10

Ingredients:

- cans black beans
- cup shredded cheddar
- can cube green chilies
- teaspoons taco seasoning
- whole wheat flour tortillas
- Olive oil

Directions:

1. Begin by preheating the toaster oven to 350°F.
2. Drain black beans and mash in a medium bowl with a fork.
3. Mix in cheese, chilies, and taco seasoning until all ingredients are thoroughly combined.
4. Evenly spread the mixture over each tortilla and wrap tightly.
5. Brush each side lightly with olive oil and place on a baking sheet.
6. Bake for 12 minutes, turn the side and bake for another 13 minutes.

Nutrition:

Calories: 367, Sodium: 136 mg,

Dietary Fiber: 14.4 g, Total Fat: 2.8 g,

Total Carbs: 64.8 g, Protein: 22.6 g.

50. Spice-Roasted Almonds

Difficulty: Easy

Preparation Time: 5 minutes

Cooking time: 10 minutes

Servings: 32

Ingredients:

- 1 tablespoon chili powder
- 1 tablespoon olive oil
- 1/2 teaspoon salt
- 1/2 teaspoon ground cumin
- 1/2 teaspoon ground coriander
- 1/4 teaspoon ground cinnamon
- 1/4 teaspoon black pepper
- cups whole almonds

Directions:

1. Begin by preheating the toaster oven to 350°F.
2. Mix olive oil, chili powder, coriander, cinnamon, cumin, salt, and pepper.
3. Add almonds and toss together.
4. Move to a baking pan and bake for 10 minutes.

Nutrition:

Calories: 39,

Sodium: 37 mg,

Dietary Fiber: 0.8 g,

Total Fat: 3.5 g,

Total Carbs: 1.4 g,

Protein: 1.3 g.

51. Sweet Potato and Parsnip Spiralized Latkes

Difficulty: Easy

Preparation Time: 20 minutes

Cooking time: 20 minutes

Servings: 12

Ingredients:

- 1 medium sweet potato
- 1 large parsnip
- cups of water
- 1 egg + 1 egg white
- scallions
- 1/2 teaspoon garlic powder
- 1/2 teaspoon sea salt
- 1/2 teaspoon ground pepper

Directions:

1 Start by spiraling the sweet potato and parsnip and chopping the scallions, reserving only the green parts.

2 Preheat toaster oven to 425°F.

3 Boil 4 cups of water. Place all of your noodles in a colander and pour the boiling water over the top, draining well.

4 Let the noodles cold, then grab handfuls, place them in a paper towel, squeeze to remove as much liquid as possible.

5 Add noodles, scallions, garlic powder, and salt, and pepper, mix well.

6 Prepare a baking sheet; scoop out 1/4 cup of the mixture at a time and place on sheet.

7 Slightly press down each scoop with your hands, then bake for 20 minutes, flipping halfway through.

Nutrition:

Calories: 24, Sodium: 91 mg,

Dietary Fiber: 1.0 g,

Total Fat: 0.4 g,

Total Carbs: 4.3 g,

Protein: 0.9 g.

52. Vegetable Egg Rolls

Difficulty: Easy

Preparation Time: 15 minutes

Cooking time: 10 minutes

Servings: 8

Ingredients:

- ½ cup chopped mushrooms
- ½ cup grated carrots
- ½ cup chopped zucchini
- green onions, chopped
- tablespoons low-sodium soy sauce
- egg roll wrappers
- 1 tablespoon cornstarch
- 1 egg, beaten

Directions:

1 Mix the mushrooms, carrots, zucchini, green onions, and soy sauce, and stir together in a medium bowl.

2 Put the egg roll wrappers on a surface.

3 Place each with about 3 tablespoons of the vegetable mixture.

4 Combine the cornstarch and egg in a small bowl.

5 Roll up the wrappers.

6 Put some of the egg mixtures on the outside of the egg rolls to seal.

7 Air-fry for 8 to 10 minutes or until the egg rolls are brown and crunchy.

Nutrition:

Calories: 112;

Total Fat: 1g;

Saturated Fat: 0g;

Cholesterol: 23mg;

Sodium: 417mg;

Carbohydrates: 21g;

Fiber: 1g;

Protein: 4g

53. Veggies on Toast

Difficulty: Easy

Preparation Time: 12 minutes

Cooking time: 11 minutes

Servings: 4

Ingredients:

- 1 red bell pepper, cut into ½-inch strips
- 1 cup sliced button or cremini mushrooms
- 1 small yellow squash, sliced
- green onions, cut into ½-inch cuts
- Extra light olive oil
- to 6 pieces sliced French bread
- tablespoons softened butter
- ½ cup soft goat cheese

Directions:

1 Mix the red pepper, mushrooms, squash, and green onions in the air fryer and mist with oil.

2 Cook for 15 minutes until the vegetables are tender, shaking the basket once during cooking time.

3 Take out the vegetables from the basket and set aside.

4 Put the bread with butter and place in the air fryer.

5 Heat up for 2 to 4 minutes or until golden brown.

6 Put the goat cheese on the toasted bread and top with the vegetables; serve warm.

Nutrition:

Calories: 162

Total Fat: 11g;

Saturated Fat: 7g;

Cholesterol: 30mg;

Sodium: 160mg;

Carbohydrates: 9g;

Fiber: 2g;

Protein: 7g

54. Jumbo Stuffed Mushrooms

Difficulty: Easy

Preparation Time: 10 minutes

Cooking time: 20 minutes

Servings: 4

Ingredients:

- jumbo Portobello mushrooms
- 1 tablespoon olive oil
- ¼ cup ricotta cheese
- tablespoons Parmesan cheese
- cup frozen chopped spinach, softened and drained
- bread crumbs
- ¼ teaspoon minced fresh rosemary

Directions:

1 Apply the mushrooms with a damp cloth.

2 Take out the stems and throw away.

3 With a spoon, lightly scrape out most of the gills.

4 Rub the mushrooms with the olive oil.

5 Place in the air fryer basket, hollow side up, and bake for 3 minutes.

6 Carefully take out the mushroom caps because they will contain liquid. Drain the liquid out of the lids.

7 Mix the ricotta, 3 tablespoons of Parmesan cheese, spinach, bread crumbs, rosemary, and mix well in a medium bowl.

8 Dash with the remaining 3 tablespoons of Parmesan cheese.

9 Place the mushroom caps back into the basket.

10 Bake for 5 to 10 minutes or until the filling is hot and the mushroom caps are tender.

Nutrition:

Calories: 117;

Total Fat: 7g;

Saturated Fat: 3g;

Cholesterol: 10mg;

Sodium: 180mg;

Carbohydrates: 8g;

Fiber: 1g;

Protein: 7g

55. Mushroom Pita Pizzas

Difficulty: Easy

Preparation Time: 10 minutes

Cooking time: 5 minutes

Servings: 4

Ingredients:

4 (3-inch) pitas

1 tablespoon olive oil

¾ cup pizza sauce

1 (4-ounce) jar sliced mushrooms, drained

½ teaspoon dried basil

2 green onions, minced

1 cup grated mozzarella or provolone cheese

1 cup sliced grape tomatoes

Directions:

Put each piece of pita with oil and top with the pizza sauce.

Put the mushrooms and sprinkle with basil and green onions. Put with the grated cheese.

Bake for 5 to 10 minutes or until the cheese is melted and starts to brown. Put with the grape tomatoes.

Nutrition:

Calories: 231; Total Fat: 9g;

Saturated Fat: 4g;

Cholesterol: 15mg;

Sodium: 500mg;

Carbohydrates: 25g;

Fiber: 2g; Protein: 13g

56. Spinach Quiche

Difficulty: Easy

Preparation Time: 10 minutes

Cooking time: 20 minutes

Servings: 3

Ingredients:

- eggs
- 1 cup frozen chopped spinach, softened and drained
- heavy cream
- tablespoons honey mustard
- ½ cup grated Swiss or Havarti cheese
- ½ teaspoon dried thyme
- Pinch salt
- Freshly ground black pepper
- Nonstick baking spray with flour

Directions:

1 Beat the eggs until blended in a medium bowl. Mix in the spinach, cream, honey mustard, cheese, thyme, salt, and pepper.

2 A baking pan with nonstick spray. Put the egg mixture into the pan.

3 Cook for 18 to 22 minutes or until the egg mixture is puffed, light golden brown, and set.

4 Leave it to cool for 5 minutes, then chop into wedges.

Nutrition:

Calories: 203;

Total Fat: 15g;

Saturated Fat: 8g;

Cholesterol: 199mg;

Sodium: 211mg;

Carbohydrates: 6g;

Fiber: 0g;

Protein: 11g

57. Yellow Squash Fritters

Difficulty: Easy

Preparation Time: 15 minutes

Cooking time: 7 minutes

Servings: 4

Ingredients:

- 1 (3-ounce) package cream cheese, softened
- 1 egg, beaten
- ½ teaspoon dried oregano

- Pinch salt
- Freshly ground black pepper
- 1 medium yellow summer squash, grated
- grated carrot
- 1 cup bread crumbs
- tablespoons olive oil

Directions:

1 Mix the cream cheese, egg, oregano, and salt and pepper in a medium bowl. Put the squash and carrot, and mix well. Place in the bread crumbs.

2 Put about 2 tablespoons of this mixture into a patty about ½ inch thick. Repeat with the remaining mixture. Brush the fritters with olive oil.

3 About 7 to 9 minutes, Air-fry until crisp and golden.

Nutrition:

Calories: 234; Total Fat: 17g;

Saturated Fat: 6g; Cholesterol: 64mg;

Sodium: 261mg;Carbohydrates: 16g;

Fiber: 2g; Protein: 6g

58. Pesto Gnocchi

Difficulty: Easy

Preparation Time: 5 minutes

Cooking time: 20 minutes

Servings: 4

Ingredients:

- 1 tablespoon olive oil
- 1 onion, finely chopped
- cloves garlic, sliced
- 1 (16-ounce) package shelf-stable gnocchi
- 1 (8-ounce) jar pesto
- 1 cup grated Parmesan cheese

Directions:

1 Mix the oil, onion, garlic, and gnocchi in a 6-by-6-by-2-inch pan and put it into the air fryer.

2 Cook for 15 minutes, then take out the pan and mix.

3 Put back the pan to the air fryer and cook for 13 minutes

4 Take out the pan from the air fryer. Place in the pesto and Parmesan cheese, and serve immediately.

Nutrition:

Calories: 646; Total Fat: 32g;

Saturated Fat: 7g; Cholesterol: 103mg;

Sodium: 461mg; Carbohydrates: 69g;

Fiber: 2g; Protein: 22g

59. English Muffin Tuna Sandwiches

Difficulty: Easy

Preparation Time: 8 minutes

Cooking time: 5 minutes

Servings: 4

Ingredients:

- 1 (6-ounce) can chunk light tuna, drained
- ¼ cup mayonnaise

- tablespoons mustard
- 1 tablespoon lemon juice
- green onions, minced
- English muffins split with a fork
- tablespoons softened butter
- thin slices provolone or Muenster cheese

Directions:

1. Mix the tuna, mayonnaise, mustard, lemon juice, and green onions in a small bowl.
2. Grease the cut side of the English muffins.
3. Cook butter-side up in the air fryer for 2 to 4 minutes or until light golden brown.
4. Take out the muffins from the air fryer basket.
5. Place each muffin with one slice of cheese and go back to the air fryer.
6. Cook for 3 to 6 minutes
7. Take out the muffins from the air fryer, top with the tuna mixture, and serve.

Nutrition:

Calories: 389;

Total Fat: 23g;

Saturated Fat: 10g;

Cholesterol: 50mg;

Sodium: 495mg;

Carbohydrates: 25g;

Fiber: 3g;

Protein: 21g

60. Tuna Zucchini Melts

Difficulty: Easy

Preparation Time: 15 minutes

Cooking time: 10 minutes

Servings: 5

Ingredients:

- corn tortillas
- tablespoons softened butter
- (6-ounce) can chunk light tuna, drained
- 1 cup mayonnaise
- tablespoons mustard
- 1 cup shredded Cheddar or Colby cheese

Directions:

1. Put softened butter in a tortilla.
2. Put in the air fryer basket and grill for 2 to 3 minutes or until the tortillas are crisp. Take out from the basket and set aside.
3. Mix the tuna, zucchini, mayonnaise, and mustard in a medium bowl.
4. Divide the tuna combination
5. Place each with some of the shredded cheese.
6. Cook in the air fryer for 2 to 4 minutes
7. Serve.

Nutrition:

Calories: 428; Total Fat: 30g;

Saturated Fat: 13g; Cholesterol: 71mg;

Sodium: 410mg; Carbohydrates: 19g;

Fiber: 3g;

Protein: 22g

61. Shrimp and Grilled Cheese Sandwiches

Difficulty: Medium

Preparation Time: 10 minutes

Cooking time: 5 minutes

Servings: 4

Ingredients:

- 1¼ cups shredded Colby, Cheddar, or Havarti cheese
- 1 (6-ounce) can tiny shrimp, drained
- tablespoons mayonnaise
- tablespoons minced green onion
- slices whole-grain or whole-wheat bread
- tablespoons softened butter

Directions:

1 Mix the cheese, shrimp, mayonnaise, and green onion in a medium bowl.

2 Put this combination on two of the slices of bread.

3 Place with the other slices of bread to make two sandwiches.

4 Cook in the oven for 5 to 7 minutes

5 Until the bread is browned and crisp and the cheese is melted.

6 Chop in half and serve warm.

Nutrition:

Calories: 276; Total Fat: 14g;

Saturated Fat: 6g; Cholesterol: 115mg;

Sodium: 573mg; Carbohydrates: 16g;

Fiber: 2g;

Protein: 22g

62. Shrimp Croquettes

Difficulty: Medium

Preparation Time: 12 minutes

Cooking time: 8 minutes

Servings: 3

Ingredients:

- cooked shrimp, shelled and deveined
- 1½ cups bread crumbs, divided
- 1 egg, beaten
- tablespoon lemon juice
- green onions, finely chopped
- ½ teaspoon dried basil
- Pinch salt
- Freshly ground black pepper
- tablespoons olive oil

Directions:

1 Finely chop the shrimp. Take about 1 tablespoon of the finely chopped shrimp and chop it further until it's almost a paste. Set aside.

2 In a medium bowl, combine ½ cup of the bread crumbs with the egg and lemon juice. Let stand for 5 minutes.

3 Combine the shrimp, green onions, basil, salt, and pepper into the bread crumb mixture.

4 Mix the remaining 1 cup of bread crumbs with the olive oil on a shallow plate; mix well.

5 Form the shrimp mixture into 1½-inch round balls and crush firmly with your hands.

6 Put in the bread crumb mixture to coat.

7 Air-fry the croquettes until they are brown and crisp.

Nutrition:

Calories: 330; Total Fat: 12g;

Saturated Fat: 2g; Cholesterol: 201mg;

Sodium: 539mg;

Carbohydrates: 31g;

Fiber: 2g;

Protein: 24g

63. Dutch Pancake with Shrimp Salsa

Difficulty: Medium

Preparation Time: 5 minutes

Cooking time: 10 minutes

Servings: 4

Ingredients:

- 1 tablespoon plus 2 teaspoons butter
- eggs
- ½ cup flour
- ½ cup milk
- teaspoon of salt
- 1 cup of salsa
- 1 cup frozen fully cooked small shrimp, thawed

Directions:

1 Preheat the air fryer with a pan.

2 Put in the butter and heat until it melts.

3 Mix the eggs, flour, milk, and salt in a medium bowl and beat well with an eggbeater until well mixed and frothy.

4 Take out the basket with the pan from the air fryer and tilt, so the butter covers the pan's bottom.

5 Place the batter into the hot pan and put it back in the fryer.

6 Cook for 12 to 16 minutes or until the pancake is puffed and golden brown.

7 Whisk together the salsa and shrimp and top the pancake with this mixture.

Nutrition:

Calories: 213;

Total Fat: 9g;

Saturated Fat: 5g;

Cholesterol: 198mg;

Sodium: 593mg;

Carbohydrates: 18g;

Fiber: 2g;

Protein: 14g

64. Steamed Scallops with Dill

Difficulty: Medium

Preparation Time: 5 minutes

Cooking time: 4 minutes

Servings: 4

Ingredients:

- 1-pound sea scallops
- 1 tablespoon lemon juice
- teaspoons olive oil

- 1 teaspoon dried dill
- Pinch salt
- Freshly ground black pepper

Directions:

1 Make sure the scallops for a small muscle attached to the side, pull it off, and discard it.

2 Mix the scallops with lemon juice, olive oil, dill, salt, and pepper. Place into the air fryer basket.

3 Steam for 5-6 minutes, until the scallops are just set when tested with your finger.

4 The internal temperature should be 150°F at a minimum.

Nutrition:

Calories: 121; Total Fat: 3g;

Saturated Fat: 0g; Cholesterol: 37mg;

Sodium: 223mg; Carbohydrates: 3g;

Fiber: 0g; Protein: 19g

65. Chicken Pita Sandwiches

Difficulty: Medium

Preparation Time: 10 minutes

Cooking time: 10 minutes

Servings: 4

Ingredients:

- boneless and skinless chicken breasts, chopped into 1-inch cubes
- 1 red onion, sliced
- 1 red bell pepper, sliced
- Italian salad dressing, divided
- ½ teaspoon dried thyme
- pita pockets, split
- cups torn butter lettuce
- 1 cup chopped cherry tomatoes

Directions:

1 Place the chicken, onion, and bell pepper in the air fryer basket. Drizzle with 1 tablespoon of the Italian salad dressing, add the thyme and toss.

2 Cook for 9 to 11 minutes

3 Move the chicken and vegetables to a bowl and toss with the remaining salad dressing.

4 Bring together sandwiches with the pita pockets, butter lettuce, and cherry tomatoes.

Nutrition:

Calories: 414; Total Fat: 19g;

Saturated Fat: 4g; Cholesterol: 101mg;

Sodium: 253mg; Carbohydrates: 22g;

Fiber: 2g; Protein: 36g

66. Chicken à la King

Difficulty: Medium

Preparation Time: 10 minutes

Cooking time: 17 minutes

Servings: 4

Ingredients:

- boneless and skinless chicken breasts, chopped
- mushrooms, sliced
- 1 red bell pepper, chopped

- 1 tablespoon olive oil
- 1 (10-ounce) package refrigerated Alfredo sauce
- ½ teaspoon dried thyme
- slices French bread
- tablespoons softened butter

Directions:

1 Put the chicken, mushrooms, and bell pepper in the air fryer basket.

2 Put with the olive oil and toss to coat.

3 Cook for 10 to 15 minutes.

4 Take the chicken and vegetables to a 6-inch metal bowl and stir in the Alfredo sauce and thyme. Go back to the air fryer and cook for 3 to 4 minutes or until hot.

5 Meanwhile, put the butter in French bread slices. When the chicken is done, take the pan from the basket and add the bread and butter-side.

6 Put the toast on a serving plate and top with the chicken.

Nutrition:

Calories: 744;

Total Fat: 32g;

Saturated Fat: 15g;

Cholesterol: 142mg;

Sodium: 3,904mg;

Carbohydrates: 64g;

Fiber: 2g;

Protein: 50g

67. Hot and Sweet Bacon and Bell Pepper Sandwiches

Difficulty: Medium

Preparation Time: 15 minutes

Cooking time: 7 minutes

Servings: 4

Ingredients:

- 1 cup spicy barbecue sauce
- tablespoons honey
- slices precooked bacon, cut into thirds
- 1 red bell pepper, sliced
- 1 yellow bell pepper, sliced
- pita pockets, cut in half
- 1¼ cups torn butter lettuce leaves
- tomatoes, sliced

Directions:

1 Mix the barbecue sauce and the honey in a small bowl. Coat this mixture lightly onto the bacon slices and the red and yellow pepper slices.

2 Place the peppers into the oven basket and grill for 5 minutes. Put in the bacon, and grill for 2 minutes or until the bacon is browned and the peppers are tender.Load the pita halves with the bacon, peppers, any remaining barbecue sauce, lettuce, tomatoes, and serve immediately.

Nutrition:

Calories: 358; Total Fat: 17g; Saturated Fat: 5g;

Cholesterol: 42mg; Sodium: 1,228mg;

Carbohydrates: 35g; Fiber: 3g; Protein: 17g

68. Air Fried Mushroom Frittata

Difficulty: Medium

Preparation Time: 8 minutes

Cooking time: 12 minutes

Servings: 2

Ingredients:

- egg whites
- 1/3 cup mushrooms, sliced
- 1 large tomato, sliced
- ¼ cup finely chopped chives
- tbsp. milk
- Salt and ground black pepper

Directions:

1 Start by setting your air fryer toast oven to 320 F.

2 Beat the egg whites and milk in a large bowl. Add in the fresh ingredients and mix until well combined, then set the bowl aside.

3 Lightly grease oven's frying pan and transfer the egg mixture into the pan.

4 Cook in the fryer for about 10 -12 minutes or until done to desire.

Nutrition:

Calories: 360 kcal

Carbs: 10.8 g,

Fat: 28.6 g,

Protein: 4.6 g.

69. French Toast from Heaven!

Difficulty: Medium

Preparation Time: 5 minutes

Cooking time: 20 minutes

Servings: 3

Ingredients:

- slices of preferred bread
- ¾ cup of milk
- eggs
- 1 tsp. pure vanilla extract
- 1 tbsp. ground cinnamon

Directions:

1 Start by preheating your air fryer toast oven at 320 degrees F.

2 Mix all the ingredients except the bread in a medium bowl until well mixed.

3 Dunk each slice of bread into the egg mix, gently shake the excess off and place it in a greased pan.

4 Cook in the fryer, each side for 3 minutes, and repeat for the remaining slices.

5 To serve, drizzle with maple syrup.

Nutrition:

Calories: 245 kcal,

Carbs: 28.5 g,

Fat: 7.5 g,

Protein: 14.9 g.

70. Crunchy Zucchini Hash Browns

Difficulty: Medium

Preparation Time: 30 minutes

Cooking time: 15 minutes

Servings: 3

Ingredients:

- medium zucchini, peeled and grated
- 1 tsp. onion powder
- 1 tsp. garlic powder
- tbsp. almond flour
- 1 ½ tsp. chili flakes
- Salt and freshly ground pepper to taste
- tsp. olive oil

Directions:

1 Put the grated zucchini in between layers of kitchen towel and squeeze to drain excess water. Pour 1 tsp of oil in a pan, preferably non-stick, over medium heat, and sauté the potatoes for about 3 minutes.

2 Transfer the zucchini to a shallow bowl and let cool. Sprinkle the zucchini with the remaining ingredients and mix until well combined.

3 Transfer the zucchini mixture to a flat plate and pat it down to make one compact layer.

4 Put in the fridge for 25 minutes.

5 Set your air fryer toast oven to 360 degrees F.

6 Meanwhile, take out the flattened zucchini and divide it into equal portions using a knife or cookie cutter.

7 Lightly brush your air fryer toast oven's basket with the remaining teaspoon of oil.

8 Gently place the zucchini pieces into the greased basket and fry for 12-15 minutes, flipping the hash browns halfway through.

9 Enjoy hot!

Nutrition:

Calories: 195 kcal,

Carbs: 10.4 g,

Fat: 13.1 g,

Protein: 9.6 g.

71. Japanese Chicken Mix

Preparation Time: 10 minutes

Cooking Time: 8 minutes

Servings: 2

Ingredients:

- chicken thighs, skinless and boneless
- ginger slices, chopped
- garlic cloves, minced
- ¼ cup soy sauce
- ¼ cup mirin
- 1/8 cup sake
- ½ teaspoon sesame oil
- 1/8 cup water
- 2 tablespoons sugar

- 1 tablespoon cornstarch mixed with 2 tablespoons water
- Sesame seeds for serving

Directions:

1 In a bowl, mix chicken thighs with ginger, garlic, soy sauce, mirin, sake, oil, water, sugar and cornstarch, toss well, transfer to preheated air fryer and cook at 360 degrees F for 8 minutes.

2 Divide among plates, sprinkle sesame seeds on top and serve with a side salad for lunch.

3 Enjoy!

Nutrition:

Calories 300,

Fat 7,

Fiber 9,

Carbs 17,

Protein 10

72. Prosciutto Sandwich

Preparation Time: 10 minutes

Cooking Time: 5 minutes

Servings: 1

Ingredients:

- bread slices
- mozzarella slices
- 2 tomato slices
- 2 prosciutto slices
- 2 basil leaves
- 1 teaspoon olive oil
- A pinch of salt and black pepper

Directions:

1 Arrange mozzarella and prosciutto on a bread slice.

2 Season with salt and pepper, place in your air fryer and cook at 400 degrees F for 5 minutes.

3 Drizzle oil over prosciutto, add tomato and basil, cover with the other bread slice, cut sandwich in half and serve.

4 Enjoy!

Nutrition:

Calories 172,

Fat 3,

Fiber 7,

Carbs 9,

Protein 5

73. Lentils Fritters

Preparation Time: 10 minutes

Cooking Time: 10 minutes

Servings: 2

Ingredients:

- 1 cup yellow lentils, soaked in water for 1 hour and drained
- 1 hot chili pepper, chopped
- 1 inch ginger piece, grated
- ½ teaspoon turmeric powder
- 1 teaspoon garam masala

- 1 teaspoon baking powder
- Salt and black pepper to the taste
- teaspoons olive oil
- 1/3 cup water
- ½ cup cilantro, chopped
- 1 and ½ cup spinach, chopped
- garlic cloves, minced
- ¾ cup red onion, chopped
- Mint chutney for serving

Directions:

1 In your blender, mix lentils with chili pepper, ginger, turmeric, garam masala, baking powder, salt, pepper, olive oil, water, cilantro, spinach, onion and garlic, blend well and shape medium balls out of this mix.

2 Place them all in your preheated air fryer at 400 degrees F and cook for 10 minutes.

3 Serve your veggie fritters with a side salad for lunch.

4 Enjoy!

Nutrition:

Calories 142,

Fat 2,

Fiber 8,

Carbs 12,

Protein 4

74. Lunch Potato Salad

Preparation Time: 10 minutes

Cooking Time: 25 minutes

Servings: 4

Ingredients:

- pound red potatoes, halved
- tablespoons olive oil
- Salt and black pepper to the taste
- 2 green onions, chopped
- 1 red bell pepper, chopped
- 1/3 cup lemon juice
- tablespoons mustard

Directions:

1 On your air fryer's basket, mix potatoes with half of the olive oil, salt and pepper and cook at 350 degrees F for 25 minutes shaking the fryer once.

2 In a bowl, mix onions with bell pepper and roasted potatoes and toss.

3 In a small bowl, mix lemon juice with the rest of the oil and mustard and whisk really well.

4 Add this to potato salad, toss well and serve for lunch.

5 Enjoy!

Nutrition:

Calories 211,

Fat 6,

Fiber 8,

Carbs 12,

Protein 4

75. Corn Casserole

Preparation Time: 10 minutes

Cooking Time: 15 minutes

Servings: 4

Ingredients:

- cups corn
- tablespoons flour
- 1 egg
- ¼ cup milk
- ½ cup light cream
- ½ cup Swiss cheese, grated
- tablespoons butter
- Salt and black pepper to the taste
- Cooking spray

Directions:

1 In a bowl, mix corn with flour, egg, milk, light cream, cheese, salt, pepper and butter and stir well.

2 Grease your air fryer's pan with cooking spray, pour cream mix, spread and cook at 320 degrees F for 15 minutes.

3 Serve warm for lunch.

4 Enjoy!

Nutrition:

Calories 281,

Fat 7,

Fiber 8,

Carbs 9,

Protein 6

76. Bacon and Garlic Pizzas

Preparation Time: 10 minutes

Cooking Time: 10 minutes

Servings: 4

Ingredients:

- dinner rolls, frozen
- garlic cloves minced
- ½ teaspoon oregano dried
- ½ teaspoon garlic powder
- 1 cup tomato sauce
- bacon slices, cooked and chopped
- 1 and ¼ cups cheddar cheese, grated
- Cooking spray

Directions:

1 Place dinner rolls on a working surface and press them to obtain 4 ovals.

2 Spray each oval with cooking spray, transfer them to your air fryer and cook them at 370 degrees F for 2 minutes.

3 Spread tomato sauce on each oval, divide garlic, sprinkle oregano and garlic powder and top with bacon and cheese.

4 Return pizzas to your heated air fryer and cook them at 370 degrees F for 8 minutes more.

5 Serve them warm for lunch. Enjoy!

Nutrition:

Calories 217, Fat 5, Fiber 8,

Carbs 12, Protein 4

77. Sweet and Sour Sausage Mix

Preparation Time: 10 minutes

Cooking Time: 10 minutes

Servings: 4

Ingredients:

- 1 pound sausages, sliced
- 1 red bell pepper, cut into strips
- ½ cup yellow onion, chopped
- tablespoons brown sugar
- 1/3 cup ketchup
- tablespoons mustard
- tablespoons apple cider vinegar
- ½ cup chicken stock

Directions:

1 In a bowl, mix sugar with ketchup, mustard, stock and vinegar and whisk well.

2 In your air fryer's pan, mix sausage slices with bell pepper, onion and sweet and sour mix, toss and cook at 350 degrees F for 10 minutes.

3 Divide into bowls and serve for lunch.

4 Enjoy!

Nutrition:

Calories 162,

Fat 6,

Fiber 9,

Carbs 12,

Protein 6

78. Meatballs and Tomato Sauce

Preparation Time: 10 minutes

Cooking Time: 15 minutes

Servings: 4

Ingredients:

- 1 pound lean beef, ground
- green onions, chopped
- garlic cloves, minced
- 1 egg yolk
- ¼ cup bread crumbs
- Salt and black pepper to the taste
- 1 tablespoon olive oil
- 16 ounces tomato sauce
- tablespoons mustard

Directions:

1 In a bowl, mix beef with onion, garlic, egg yolk, bread crumbs, salt and pepper, stir well and shape medium meatballs out of this mix.

2 Grease meatballs with the oil, place them in your air fryer and cook them at 400 degrees F for 10 minutes.

3 In a bowl, mix tomato sauce with mustard, whisk, add over meatballs, toss them and cook at 400 degrees F for 5 minutes more.

4 Divide meatballs and sauce on plates and serve for lunch.

5 Enjoy!

Nutrition:

Calories 300, Fat 8, Fiber 9,

Carbs 16, Protein 5

79. Crunchy Hash Browns

Difficulty: Hard

Preparation Time: 15 minutes

Cooking time: 7 minutes

Servings: 4

Ingredients:

- medium potatoes, peeled and grated
- 1 tsp. onion powder
- 1 tsp. garlic powder
- tbsp. cornflour
- 1 ½ tsp. chili flakes
- Salt and freshly ground pepper to taste
- 1 tsp. olive oil

Directions:

1 Put the chopped potatoes in a large bowl

2 Cover with ice-cold water and let it sit for a minute.

3 Drain the water and repeat this step two times. (This helps in eliminating the excess starch)

4 Pour 1 teaspoon of oil in a pan, preferably non-stick, over medium heat, and sauté the potatoes for about 3 minutes.

5 Move the potatoes to a shallow bowl and let cool. Sprinkle the potatoes with the remaining ingredients and mix until well combined.

6 Transfer the potato mix to a flat plate and pat it down to make one compact layer. Place in the fridge for 20 minutes.

7 Set your air fryer toast oven to 360 degrees F.

8 Meanwhile, take out the flattened potato and divide it into equal portions using a knife or cookie cutter.

9 Lightly brush your air fryer toast oven's basket with the remaining teaspoon of olive oil.

10 Gently place the potato pieces into the greased basket and fry for 12-15 minutes, flipping the hash browns halfway through.

11 Enjoy hot!

Nutrition:

Calories: 295 kcal,

Carbs: 60.9 g,

Fat: 3.7 g,

Protein: 6.6 g.

80. Meaty Breakfast Omelet

Difficulty: Hard

Preparation Time: 10 minutes

Cooking time: 10 minutes

Servings: 2

Ingredients:

- large eggs
- 100g ham, cut into small pieces
- ¼ cup milk
- ¾ cup mixed vegetables (mushrooms, scallions, bell pepper)
- ¼ cup mixed cheddar and mozzarella cheese

- 1 tsp. mixed herbs
- Salt and freshly ground pepper to taste

Directions:

1 Mix the milk and eggs in a bowl

2 Add in the remaining ingredients apart from the cheese and mixed herbs and beat well using a fork.

3 Pour the egg mixture into an evenly greased pan, then place it in the basket of your air fryer toast oven.

4 Cook for 20 minutes at 350 degrees F

5 Sprinkle the cheese and mixed herbs on the omelet halfway through cook time.

6 Gently loosen the omelet from the sides of the pan using a spatula.

7 Serve hot!

Nutrition:

Calories: 278 kcal,

Carbs: 1.3 g,

Fat: 4.6 g,

Protein: 24.1 g.

81. Ham and Cheese sandwich

Difficulty: Very Hard

Preparation Time: 15 minutes

Cooking time: 20 minutes

Servings: 2

Ingredients:

- eggs
- slices of bread of choice
- slices turkey
- slices ham
- tbsp. half and half cream
- tsp. melted butter
- slices Swiss cheese
- ¼ tsp. pure vanilla extract
- Powdered sugar and raspberry jam for serving

Directions:

1 Combine the eggs, vanilla, and cream in a bowl and set aside.

2 Make a sandwich with the bread layered with cheese slice, turkey, ham, cheese slice, and the top slice of bread to make two sandwiches. Gently press on the sandwiches to somewhat flatten them.

3 Set your air fryer toast oven to 350 degrees F.

4 Spread out kitchen aluminum foil, cut it about the same size as the sandwich, and spread the melted butter on the foil's surface.

5 Dip the sandwich in the egg mixture and let it soak for about 20 seconds on each side. Repeat this for the other sandwich. Place the soaked sandwiches on the prepared foil sheets, then place them on the basket in your fryer.

6 Cook for 12 minutes, then flip the sandwiches and brush with the remaining butter and cook for another 5 minutes or until well browned.

7 Place the cooked sandwiched on a plate and top with the powdered sugar, and serve with a small raspberry jam bowl.

Nutrition:

Calories: 735 kcal,

Carbs: 13.4 g,

Fat: 47.9 g,

Protein: 40.8 g.

82. Classic Fish and Chips

Difficulty: Very Hard

Preparation Time: 15 minutes

Cooking time: 30 minutes

Servings: 4

Ingredients:

- 450g tilapia/ catfish/ cod fillet
- russet potatoes, peeled and cut into French fries (or wedges)
- tbsp. vegetable oil
- 1 egg
- 1 cup panko breadcrumbs
- ¼ cup all-purpose flour
- 1 tbsp. sea salt
- Ground pepper to taste

Directions:

1 Toss the prepared potatoes with half the salt, oil, and pepper, if desired.

2 Set your air fryer toast oven to 400 degrees F and cook the potatoes for 15-20 minutes, shaking halfway through to ensure they cook evenly and don't burn.

3 As the potatoes cook, put the flour in a shallow bowl, beat the egg, put in a second bowl, and in a third bowl the panko crumbs.

4 Dredge the fillet pieces, one a time, in the flour, egg, and panko.

5 Cook the fish for 15 minutes at 330 degrees F, flipping halfway through cook time.

6 Serve hot with your favorite sauces. Enjoy!

Nutrition:

Calories: 307 kcal,

Carbs: 31.2 g,

Fat: 9.1 g,

Protein: 25.8 g.

CHAPTER 6:

Dinner

83. Cheeseburger Egg Rolls

Difficulty: Very Easy

Preparation Time: 10 minutes

Cooking time: 7 minutes

Servings: 6

Ingredients:

- egg roll wrappers
- chopped dill pickle chips
- 1 tbsp. yellow mustard
- tbsp. cream cheese
- tbsp. shredded cheddar cheese
- ½ C. chopped onion
- ½ C. chopped bell pepper
- ¼ tsp. onion powder
- ¼ tsp. garlic powder
- ounces of raw lean ground beef

Directions:

1 In a skillet, add the spices, meat, onion, and bell pepper. Stir and mash the flesh until it is fully cooked and the vegetables are soft.

2 Remove skillet from heat and add cream cheese, mustard, and cheddar cheese, stirring until melted.

3 Pour the meat mixture into a bowl and add the pickles.

4 Place egg wrappers and spoon 1/6 of the meat mixture into each. Dampen the edges of the egg roll with water. Fold the sides in half and seal with water.

5 Repeat with all the other egg rolls.

6 Place the rolls in a deep fryer, one batch at a time.

7 Place the air fryer Rack on the middle-shelf. Set temperature to 391°F, and set time to 7 minutes.

Nutrition:

Calories 153 Fat 4 g Protein 12 g Sugar 3 g

84. Air Fried Grilled Steak

Difficulty: Very Easy

Preparation Time: 5 minutes

Cooking time: 45 minutes

Servings: 2

Ingredients:

- Top sirloin steaks
- Tablespoons butter, melted
- tablespoons olive oil
- Salt and pepper to taste

Directions:

1 Preheat the Smart Air Fryer for 5 minutes.

2 Season the sirloin steaks with olive oil, salt, and pepper.

3 Place the beef in the air fryer oven basket.

4 Cook for 45 minutes at 350°F.

5 Once cooked, serve with butter.

Nutrition:

Calories 1536 Fat 123.7 g Protein 103.4 g

85. Juicy Cheeseburgers

Difficulty: Very Easy

Preparation Time: 5 minutes

Cooking time: 15 minutes

Servings: 4

Ingredients:

- 1 pound 93% lean ground beef
- 1 teaspoon Worcestershire sauce
- 1 tablespoon burger seasoning
- Salt
- Pepper
- Cooking oil
- Slices cheese
- Buns

Directions:

1 Mix the ground beef, Worcestershire, hamburger seasoning, salt, and pepper in a bowl to taste until well combined. Spray the fryer basket with cooking oil. You will only need a quick spray because hamburgers produce oil while they cook. Form 4 patties with the mixture. Place the burgers in the deep fryer. Burgers should fit without having to be stacked, but stacking is sufficient if necessary.

2 Place on the oven rack/basket.

3 Put the rack on the middle shelf of the Smart Air Fryer.

4 Put the temperature to 375 ° F and set the time to 8 minutes. Cook for 8 minutes. Open the fryer and flip the patties—Cook for 3 to 4 more minutes. Check the inside of the patties to see if they have finished cooking. You can stick a knife or fork in the center to examine the color.

5 Fill each burger with a slice of cheese. Cook for one more minute or until cheese is melted. Serve on buns with any additional toppings of your choice.

Nutrition:

Calories 566 Fat 39 g

Protein 29 g Fiber 1 g

86. Spicy Thai Beef Stir-Fry

Difficulty: Very Easy

Preparation Time: 15 minutes

Cooking time: 9 minutes

Servings: 4

Ingredients:

- 1-pound sirloin steaks, thinly sliced
- Tablespoons lime juice, divided

- 1 cup crunchy peanut butter
- ½ cup beef broth
- 1 tablespoon olive oil
- 1½ cups broccoli florets
- Cloves garlic, sliced
- 1 to 2 red chili peppers, sliced

Directions:

1 Mix the steak with 1 tablespoon of the lime juice in a bowl. Set aside.

2 Combine the peanut butter and beef broth in a small bowl and mix well. Drain the beef and add the juice from the bowl into the peanut butter mixture.

3 In a 6-inch metal bowl, combine the olive oil, steak, and broccoli.

4 Pour into the Oven rack/basket. Place the air fryer Rack on the middle-shelf of the Smart Air Fryer Oven. Set temperature to 375°F, and set time to 4 minutes.

5 Cook for 6 more minutes or until the steak is almost cooked and the broccoli is crisp and tender, shaking the basket once during cooking time.

6 Add the garlic, chili peppers, and the peanut butter mixture and stir.

7 Cook for 6 more minutes until the sauce is bubbling, and the broccoli is tender.

8 Serve over hot rice.

Nutrition:

Calories 387 Fat 22 gProtein 42 g

Fiber 2 g

87. Beef Brisket Recipe from Texas

Difficulty: Very Easy

Preparation Time: 15 minutes

Cooking time: 1 hour 30 minutes

Servings: 8

Ingredients:

- 1 ½ cup beef stock
- 1 bay leaf
- 1 tablespoon garlic powder
- 1 tablespoon onion powder
- Pounds beef brisket, trimmed
- tablespoons chili powder
- teaspoons dry mustard
- Tablespoons olive oil
- Salt and pepper to taste

Directions:

1 Preheat the Air Fryer Oven for 5 minutes.

2 All ingredients in a deep baking dish that will fit in the air fryer.

3 Bake for 1 hour and 30 minutes at 400°F.

4 Stir the beef every after 30 minutes to soak in the sauce.

Nutrition:

Calories 306

Fat 24.1 g

Protein 18.3 g

88. Copycat Taco Bell Crunch Wraps

Difficulty: Very Easy

Preparation Time: 10 minutes

Cooking time: 2 minutes

Servings: 6

Ingredients:

- Wheat tostadas
- C. sour cream
- C. Mexican blend cheese
- C. shredded lettuce
- ounces' low-sodium nacho cheese
- Roma tomatoes
- 12-inch wheat tortillas
- 1 1/3 C. water
- packets low-sodium taco seasoning
- 2 pounds of lean ground beef

Directions:

1 Ensure your air fryer is preheated to 400 degrees.

2 Make beef according to taco seasoning packets.

3 Place 2/3 C. prepared beef, 4 tbsp. Cheese, 1 tostada, 1/3 C. sour cream, 1/3 C. lettuce, 1/6th of tomatoes, and 1/3 C. cheese on each tortilla.

4 Fold up tortillas edges and repeat with remaining ingredients.

5 Lay the folded sides of tortillas down into the air fryer and spray with olive oil.

6 Set temperature to 400°F, and set time to 2 minutes. Cook 2 minutes until browned.

Nutrition:

Calories 311

Fat 9g

Protein 22g

Sugar 2g

89. Steak and Mushroom Gravy

Difficulty: Very Easy

Preparation Time: 15 minutes

Cooking time: 15 minutes

Servings: 4

Ingredients:

- Cubed steaks
- large eggs
- 1/2 dozen mushrooms
- Tablespoons unsalted butter
- Tablespoons black pepper
- tablespoons salt
- 1/2 teaspoon onion powder
- 1/2 teaspoon garlic powder
- 1/4 teaspoon cayenne powder
- 1 1/4 teaspoons paprika
- 1 1/2 cups whole milk
- 1/3 cup flour
- Tablespoons vegetable oil

Directions:

1. Combine 1/2 flour and a pinch of black pepper in a shallow bowl or on a plate.
2. Beat 2 eggs in a bowl with a pinch of salt and pepper.
3. In another shallow bowl, mix the other half of the flour with pepper to taste, garlic powder, paprika, cayenne, and onion powder.
4. Chop the mushrooms and reserve.
5. Squeeze the fillet into the first bowl of flour, then dip it into the egg and then press the fillet into the second bowl of flour until completely covered.
6. Place on the oven rack/basket.
7. Put the rack of the Smart Air Fryer on the middle shelf.
8. Set the temperature to 360 ° F and set the time to 15 minutes by turning it halfway.
9. Over medium heat, heat the butter and put in the mushrooms to the stir-fry.
10. Add 4 tablespoons of flour and pepper to the skillet and mix until there are no flour lumps.
11. Mix in whole milk and simmer.

Nutrition:

Calories 442

Fat 27 g

Protein 32 g

Fiber 2.3 g

90. Air Fryer Beef Casserole

Difficulty: Easy

Preparation Time: 5 minutes

Cooking time: 30 minutes

Servings: 4

Ingredients:

- 1 green bell pepper, seeded and chopped
- 1 onion, chopped
- 1-pound ground beef
- Cloves of garlic, minced
- Tablespoons olive oil
- Cups eggs, beaten
- Salt and pepper to taste

Directions:

1. Preheat the Smart Air Fryer oven for 5 minutes.
2. A skillet that will fit in the deep fryer combines the ground beef, onion, garlic, olive oil, and pepper—season with salt and pepper to taste.
3. Add the beaten eggs and mix well.
4. Place the plate with the meat and egg mixture in the deep fryer.
5. Place on the oven rack/basket.
6. Put the rack of the Smart Air Fryer on the middle shelf.
7. Set the temperature to 325 ° F and set the time to 30 minutes. Bake for 30 minutes.

Nutrition:

Calories 1520 Fat 125.11 g

Protein 87.9 g

91. Meat Lovers' Pizza

Difficulty: Easy

Preparation Time: 10 minutes

Cooking time: 12 minutes

Servings: 2

Ingredients:

- 1 pre-prepared 7-inch pizza crust, defrosted if necessary
- 1/3 cup of marinara sauce.
- 2 ounces of grilled steak, sliced into bite-sized pieces
- 3 ounces of salami, sliced fine
- 2 ounces of pepperoni, sliced fine
- 1/4 cup of American cheese
- ¼ cup of shredded mozzarella cheese

Directions:

1. Preheat the Smart Air Fryer Oven to 350 degrees. Lay the pizza dough flat on a sheet of parchment paper or tin foil, cut large enough to hold the entire pie crust but small enough that it will leave the edges of the air frying basket uncovered to allow for air circulation.
2. Using a fork, stab the pizza dough several times across the surface – piercing the pie crust will allow air to circulate throughout the crust and ensure even cooking.
3. With a deep soup spoon, scoop the marinara sauce onto the pizza dough and spread evenly in expanding circles over the pie-crust surface. Be sure to leave at least ½ inch of bare dough around the edges to ensure that extra-crispy crunchy first bite of the crust!
4. Distribute the steak pieces and the slices of salami and pepperoni evenly over the sauce-covered dough, then sprinkle the cheese in an even layer on top.
5. Set the air fryer timer to 12 minutes, and place the pizza with foil or paper on the fryer's basket surface. Again, be sure to leave the edges of the basket uncovered to allow for proper air circulation, and don't let your bare fingers touch the hot surface.
6. After 12 minutes, when the Smart Air Fryer Oven shuts off, the cheese should be perfectly melted and lightly crisped, and the pie crust should be golden brown. If necessary, using a spatula – or two, remove the pizza from the air fryer basket and set on a serving plate.
7. Wait a few minutes until the pie is cool enough to handle, then cut into slices and serve.

Nutrition:

Calories 342 Fat 17 g Protein 12 g Fiber 4.3 g

92. Chimichurri Skirt Steak

Difficulty: Easy

Preparation Time: 10 minutes

Cooking time: 8 minutes

Servings: 2

Ingredients:

Skirt Steak

1 cup finely chopped parsley

¼ cup finely chopped mint

2 tbsp. fresh oregano (washed & finely chopped)

Finely chopped cloves of garlic

1 tsp red pepper flakes (Crushed)

1 tbsp. ground cumin

1 tsp cayenne pepper

2 tsp smoked paprika

1 tsp salt

¼ tsp pepper

¾ cup oil

Tbsp. red wine vinegar

Directions:

Throw all the ingredients in a bowl (besides the steak) and mix well.

Put ¼ cup of the mixture in a plastic baggie with the steak and leave in the fridge overnight (2–24hrs).

Leave the bag out at room temperature for at least 30 min before popping in to the air fryer. Preheat for a minute or two to 390° F before cooking until med–rare (8–10 min).

Set temperature to 390°F, and set time to 10 minutes.

Put 2 tablespoons of the chimichurri mix on top of each steak before serving.

Nutrition:

Calories 272

Fat 3 g

Protein 32 g

Fiber 2.8 g

93. Country Fried Steak

Difficulty: Easy

Preparation Time: 5 minutes

Cooking time: 12 minutes

Servings: 2

Ingredients:

- 1 tsp. pepper
- C. almond milk
- tbsp. almond flour
- Ounces ground sausage meat
- 1 tsp. pepper
- 1 tsp. salt
- 1 tsp. garlic powder
- 1 tsp. onion powder
- 1 C. panko breadcrumbs
- 1 C. almond flour
- Beaten eggs
- Ounces sirloin steak pounded till thin

Directions:

- Season panko breadcrumbs with spices.
- Dredge steak in flour, then egg, and then seasoned panko mixture.
- Place into the air fryer basket.
- Set temperature to 370°F, and set time to 12 minutes.
- To make sausage gravy, cook sausage and drain off fat, but reserve 2 tablespoons.
- Add flour to sausage and mix until incorporated. Gradually mix in milk over

medium to high heat until it becomes thick.

- Season mixture with pepper and cook 3 minutes longer.
- Serve steak topped with gravy and enjoy.

Nutrition:

Calories 395

Fat 11 g

Protein 39 g

Sugar 5 g

94. Creamy Burger & Potato Bake

Difficulty: Easy

Preparation Time: 5 minutes

Cooking time: 55 minutes

Servings: 3

Ingredients:

1 Salt to taste

2 Freshly ground pepper, to taste

3 1/2 (10.75 ounces) can of condensed cream of mushroom soup

4 1/2-pound lean ground beef

5 1-1/2 cups peeled and thinly sliced potatoes

6 1/2 cup shredded cheddar cheese

7 1/4 cup chopped onion

8 1/4 cup and 2 tablespoons milk

Directions:

1 Lightly grease the baking pan of the air fryer. Add ground beef. For 10 minutes, cook at 360°F. Stir and crumble halfway through cooking time.

2 Meanwhile, in a bowl, whisk well pepper, salt, milk, onion, and mushroom soup. Mix well.

3 Drain fat off ground beef and transfer beef to a plate.

4 In the same air fryer baking pan, layer ½ of potatoes on the bottom, then ½ of soup mixture, and then ½ of beef. Repeat process.

5 Cover pan with foil.

6 Cook for 30 minutes.

7 Take out the aluminum foil and cook for another 15 minutes or until potatoes are tender.

8 Serve and enjoy.

Nutrition:

Calories 399

Fat 26.9 g

Protein 22.1 g

95. Beefy 'n Cheesy Spanish Rice Casserole

Difficulty: Easy

Preparation Time: 10 minutes

Cooking time: 50 minutes

Servings: 3

Ingredients:

- Tablespoons chopped green bell pepper
- 1 tablespoon chopped fresh cilantro
- 1/2-pound lean ground beef

- 1/2 cup water
- 1/2 teaspoon salt
- 1/2 teaspoon brown sugar
- 1/2 pinch ground black pepper
- 1/3 cup uncooked long-grain rice
- 1/4 cup finely chopped onion
- 1/4 cup chili sauce
- 1/4 teaspoon ground cumin
- 1/4 teaspoon Worcestershire sauce
- 1/4 cup shredded Cheddar cheese
- 1/2 (14.5 ounces) can canned tomatoes

Directions:

1 Lightly grease the baking pan with cooking spray. Add ground beef.

2 For 10 minutes, cook at 360°F. Halfway through cooking time, stir and crumble beef. Discard excess fat.

3 Stir in pepper, Worcestershire sauce, cumin, brown sugar, salt, chili sauce, rice, water, tomatoes, green bell pepper, and onion. Mix well. Cover pan with foil and cook for 25 minutes. Stirring occasionally.

4 Give it one last good stir, press down firmly, and sprinkle cheese on top.

5 Cook uncovered for 15 minutes at 390°F until tops are lightly browned.

6 Serve and enjoy with chopped cilantro.

Nutrition:

Calories 346 Fat: 19.1 g Protein 18.5 g

96. Warming Winter Beef with Celery

Difficulty: Easy

Preparation Time: 5 minutes

Cooking time: 12 minutes

Servings: 4

Ingredients:

9 ounces' tender beef, chopped

1/2 cup leeks, chopped

1/2 cup celery stalks, chopped

Cloves garlic smashed

Tablespoons red cooking wine

3/4 cup cream of celery soup

2 sprigs rosemary, chopped

1/4 teaspoon smoked paprika

3/4 teaspoons salt

Salt

1/4 teaspoon black pepper

Directions:

Add the beef, leeks, celery, and garlic to the baking dish; cook for about 5 minutes at 390 degrees F.

Once the meat is starting to tender, pour in the wine and soup—season with rosemary, smoked paprika, salt, and black pepper. Now, cook an additional 7 minutes.

Nutrition:

Calories 312Fat 17 g

Protein 22 g

Fiber 32 g

97. Beef & Veggie Spring Rolls

Difficulty: Easy

Preparation Time: 5 minutes

Cooking time: 12 minutes

Servings: 10

Ingredients:

- 2-ounce Asian rice noodles
- 1 tablespoon sesame oil
- 7-ounce ground beef
- 1 small onion, chopped
- 1 garlic cloves, crushed
- 1 cup of fresh mixed vegetables
- 1 teaspoon soy sauce
- 1 packet spring roll skins
- Tablespoons water
- Olive oil, as required

Directions:

1 Soak the noodles in warm water till it becomes soft.

2 Drain and cut into small lengths. In a pan, heat the oil and add the onion and garlic and sauté for about 4-5 minutes.

3 Add beef and cook for about 4-5 minutes.

4 Add vegetables and cook for about 5-7 minutes or till cooked through.

5 Stir in soy sauce and remove from the heat.

6 Immediately, stir in the noodles and keep aside till all the juices have been absorbed.

7 Preheat the Smart Air Fryer Oven to 350 degrees F.

8 Place the spring rolls skin onto a smooth surface.

9 Add a line of the filling diagonally across.

10 Fold the top point over the filling and then fold in both sides.

11 On the final point, brush it with water before rolling to seal.

12 Brush the spring rolls with oil.

13 Arrange the rolls in batches in the air fryer and cook for about 8 minutes.

14 Repeat with remaining rolls. Now, place spring rolls onto a baking sheet.

15 Bake for about 6 minutes per side.

Nutrition:

Calories 532

Fat 8 g

Protein 31 g

Fiber 12.3 g

98. Honey Glazed Salmon

Difficulty: Medium

Preparation Time: 10 minutes

Cooking Time: 8 minutes

Servings: 2

Ingredients:

- (6-oz.) salmon fillets
- Salt, as required
- tablespoons honey

Directions:

1 Sprinkle the salmon fillets with salt and then coat with honey.

2 Settle on the temperature at 355 degrees F.

3 When the unit beeps to show that it is preheated, open the lid.

4 Arrange the salmon fillets in an "Air Fry Basket" and place them in the oven.

5 Serve hot.

Nutrition:

Calories 289

Total Fat 10.5 g

Saturated Fat 1.5 g

Cholesterol 75 mg

Sodium 153 mg

Total Carbs 17.3 g

Fiber 0 g

Sugar 17.3 g

Protein 33.1 g

99. Sweet & Sour Glazed Salmon

Difficulty: Medium

Preparation Time: 12 minutes

Cooking Time: 20 minutes

Servings: 2

Ingredients:

- 1/3 cup soy sauce
- 1/3 cup honey
- teaspoons rice wine vinegar
- 1 teaspoon water
- (3½-oz.) salmon fillets

Directions:

1 Combine the soy sauce, honey, vinegar, and water in a medium bowl.

2 In another small bowl, reserve about half of the mixture.

3 Add salmon fillets in the remaining mixture and coat well.

4 Cover the bowl and refrigerate to marinate for about 2 hours.

5 When the unit beeps to show that it is preheated, open the lid.

6 Assemble the salmon fillets in a greased "Air Fry Basket" and insert them in the oven.

7 Flip the salmon fillets once halfway through and coat with the reserved marinade after every 3 minutes.

8 Serve hot.

Nutrition:

Calories 462

Total Fat 12.3 g

Saturated Fat 1.8 g

Cholesterol 88 mg

Sodium 2400 mg

Total Carbs 49.8 g

Fiber 0.5 g

Sugar 47.1 g

Protein 41.3 g

100. Salmon Parcel

Difficulty: Medium

Preparation Time: 15 minutes

Cooking Time: 23 minutes

Servings: 2

Ingredients:

- (4-oz.) salmon fillets
- asparagus stalks
- ¼ cup white sauce
- 1 teaspoon oil
- ¼ cup champagne
- Salt and ground black pepper, as required

Directions:

1. Combine all the ingredients.
2. Divide the salmon mixture over 2 pieces of foil evenly.
3. Seal the foil around the salmon mixture to form the packet.
4. Set the cooking time to 13 minutes.
5. When the unit beeps to show that it is preheated, open the lid.
6. Arrange the salmon parcels in "Air Fry Basket" and insert them in the oven.
7. Serve hot.

Nutrition:

Calories 243 Total Fat 12.7 g

Saturated Fat 2.2 g Cholesterol 52 mg

Sodium 240 mg Total Carbs 9.4 g

Fiber 1.8 g Sugar 6.2 g

Protein 25 g

101. Salmon with Broccoli

Difficulty: Medium

Preparation Time: 15 minutes

Cooking Time: 12 minutes

Servings: 2

Ingredients:

- 1½ cups small broccoli florets
- tablespoons vegetable oil, divided
- Salt and ground black pepper, as required
- 1 (½-inch) piece fresh ginger, grated
- 1 tablespoon soy sauce
- 1 teaspoon rice vinegar
- 1 teaspoon light brown sugar
- ¼ teaspoon cornstarch
- (6-oz.) skin-on salmon fillets
- 1 scallion, thinly sliced

Directions:

1. Combine the broccoli, 1 tablespoon of oil, salt, and black pepper in a bowl.
2. In another bowl, mix well the ginger, soy sauce, vinegar, sugar, and cornstarch.
3. Coat the salmon fillets with remaining oil and then with the ginger mixture.
4. When the unit beeps to show that it is preheated, open the lid.
5. Arrange the broccoli florets in a greased "Air Fry Basket" and top with the salmon fillets.
6. Insert the basket in the oven.

7 Serve hot.

Nutrition:

Calories 385

Total Fat 24.4 g

Saturated Fat 4.2 g

Cholesterol 75 mg

Sodium 550 mg

Total Carbs 7.8 g

Fiber 2.1 g

Sugar 3 g

Protein 35.6 g

102. Salmon with Prawns & Pasta

Difficulty: Medium

Preparation Time: 20 minutes

Cooking Time: 18 minutes

Servings: 4

Ingredients:

- 14 oz. pasta (of your choice)
- tablespoons pesto, divided
- (4-oz.) salmon steaks
- tablespoons olive oil
- ½ lb. cherry tomatoes, chopped
- large prawns, peeled and deveined
- tablespoons fresh lemon juice
- tablespoons fresh thyme, chopped

Directions:

1. Put in the pasta in a pan of salted boiling water, and cook for about 8-10 minutes or until desired doneness.
2. Meanwhile, at the bottom of a baking pan, spread 1 tablespoon of pesto.
3. Place salmon steaks and tomatoes over pesto in a single layer and drizzle with the oil.
4. Arrange the prawns on top in a single layer.
5. Drizzle with lemon juice and sprinkle with thyme.
6. Push the Time button and again turn the dial to set the cooking time to 8 minutes.
7. When the unit beeps to show that it is preheated, open the lid.
8. Arrange the baking pan in "Air Fry Basket" and insert it in the oven.
9. Drain the pasta and move into a large bowl.
10. Add the remaining pesto and toss to coat well.
11. Divide the pasta onto a serving plate and top with salmon mixture.
12. Serve immediately.

Nutrition:

Calories 592 Total Fat 23.2 g

Saturated Fat 3.8 g Cholesterol 149 mg

Sodium 203 mg Total Carbs 58.7 g

Fiber 1.5 g Sugar 2.7 g

Protein 37.9 g

103. Salmon Burgers

Difficulty: Medium

Preparation Time: 20 minutes

Cooking Time: 22 minutes

Servings: 6

Ingredients:

- large russet potatoes, peeled and cubed
- 1 (6-oz.) cooked salmon fillet
- 1 egg
- ¾ cup frozen vegetables (of your choice), parboiled and drained
- tablespoons fresh parsley, chopped
- 1 teaspoon fresh dill, chopped
- Salt and ground black pepper, as required
- 1 cup breadcrumbs
- ¼ cup olive oil

Directions:

1 In a pan of the boiling water, cook the potatoes for about 10 minutes.

2 Drain the potatoes well.

3 Move the potatoes into a bowl and mash with a potato masher.

4 Set aside to cool completely.

5 In another bowl, add the salmon and flake with a fork.

6 Add the cooked potatoes, egg, parboiled vegetables, parsley, dill, salt, and black pepper and mix until well combined.

7 Make 6 equal-sized patties from the mixture.

8 Coat patties with breadcrumb evenly and then drizzle with the oil evenly.

9 When the unit beeps to show that it is preheated, open the lid.

10 Organize the patties in "Air Fry Basket" and put it in the oven.

11 Flip the patties once halfway through.

12 Serve hot.

Nutrition:

Calories 334

Total Fat 12.1 g

Saturated Fat 2 g

Cholesterol 40 mg

Sodium 175 mg

Total Carbs 45.2 g

Fiber 6.3 g

Sugar 4 g

Protein 12.5 g

104. Ranch Tilapia

Difficulty: Medium

Preparation Time: 15 minutes

Cooking Time: 13 minutes

Servings: 4

Ingredients:

- ¾ cup cornflakes, crushed
- 1 (1-oz.) packet dry ranch-style dressing mix
- 2½ tablespoons vegetable oil
- eggs
- (6-oz.) tilapia fillets

Directions:

1 In a shallow bowl, beat the eggs.

2 In another bowl, add the cornflakes, ranch dressing, and oil and mix until a crumbly mixture forms.

3 Dip the fish fillets into the egg and then coat with the breadcrumbs mixture.

4 When the unit beeps to show that it is preheated, open the lid.

5 Arrange the tilapia fillets in a greased "Air Fry Basket" and insert it in the oven.

6 Serve hot.

Nutrition:

Calories 267

Total Fat 12.2 g

Saturated Fat 3 g

Cholesterol 1685 mg

Sodium 168 mg

Total Carbs 5.1 g

Fiber 0.2 g

Sugar 0.9 g

Protein 34.9 g

105. Chinese Cod

Difficulty: Hard

Preparation Time: 15 minutes

Cooking Time: 15 minutes

Servings: 2

Ingredients:

- (7-oz.) cod fillets
- Salt and ground black pepper, as required
- ¼ teaspoon sesame oil
- 1 cup of water
- little squares of rock sugar
- tablespoons light soy sauce
- 1 teaspoon dark soy sauce
- scallions (green part), sliced
- ¼ cup fresh cilantro, chopped
- tablespoons olive oil
- ginger slices

Directions:

1 Season each cod fillet evenly with salt and black pepper and drizzle with sesame oil.

2 Set aside at room temperature for about 15-20 minutes.

3 Dip the fish fillets into the egg and then coat with the breadcrumbs mixture.

4 When the unit beeps to show that it is preheated, open the lid.

5 Arrange the cod fillets in a greased "Air Fry Basket" and insert it in the oven.

6 Put in the water and bring it to a boil in a small pan.

7 Put in the rock sugar and both soy sauces and cook until sugar is dissolved, stirring continuously.

8 Remove from the heat and set aside.

9 Remove the cod fillets from the oven and transfer onto serving plates.

10 Top each fillet with scallion and cilantro.

11 In a small pan with oil, sauté the ginger slices for about 2-3 minutes.

12 Take out the frying pan from heat and discard the ginger slices.

13 Carefully pour the hot oil evenly over cod fillets.

14 Top with the sauce mixture and serve.

Nutrition:

Calories 380 Total Fat 23.4 g

Saturated Fat 3.1 g Cholesterol 97 mg

Sodium 2400 mg Total Carbs 5 g

Fiber 0.8 g

Sugar 1.1 g

Protein 38.3 g

106. Cod Parcel

Difficulty: Hard

Preparation Time: 20 minutes

Cooking Time: 15 minutes

Servings: 2

Ingredients:

- tablespoons butter, melted
- 1 tablespoon fresh lemon juice
- ½ teaspoon dried tarragon
- Salt and ground black pepper, as required
- ½ cup red bell peppers, seeded and thinly chopped
- ½ cup carrots, peeled and julienned
- ½ cup fennel bulbs, julienned
- (5-oz.) frozen cod fillets, thawed
- 1 tablespoon olive oil

Directions:

1 In a large bowl, mix the butter, lemon juice, tarragon, salt, and black pepper.

2 Add the bell pepper, carrot, and fennel bulb and generously coat with the mixture.

3 Arrange 2 large parchment squares onto a smooth surface.

4 Coat the cod fillets with oil and then sprinkle evenly with salt and black pepper.

5 Arrange 1 cod fillet onto each parchment square and top each evenly with the vegetables.

6 Top with any remaining sauce from the bowl.

7 Fold the parchment paper and crimp the sides to secure fish and vegetables.

8 Press the "Start/Pause" button to start.

9 When the unit beeps to show that it is preheated, open the lid.

10 Arrange the cod parcels in "Air Fry Basket" and insert it in the oven.

11 Serve hot.

Nutrition:

Calories 306 Total Fat 20 g

Saturated Fat 8.4 g Cholesterol 100 mg

Sodium 281 mg Total Carbs 6.8 g

Fiber 1.8 g Sugar 3 g Protein 26.3 g

107. Cod Burgers

Difficulty: Hard

Preparation Time: 15 minutes

Cooking Time: 7 minutes

Servings: 6

Ingredients:

- ½ lb. cod fillets
- ½ teaspoon fresh lime zest, grated finely
- ½ egg
- ½ teaspoon red chili paste
- Salt, to taste
- ½ tablespoon fresh lime juice
- tablespoons coconut, grated and divided
- 1 small scallion, chopped finely
- 1 tablespoon fresh parsley, chopped

Directions:

1 In a food processor, add cod filets, lime zest, egg, chili paste, salt, and lime juice and pulse until smooth.

2 Transfer the cod mixture into a bowl.

3 Add 1½ tablespoons coconut, scallion, and parsley and mix until well combined.

4 Make 6 equal-sized patties from the mixture.

5 In a shallow dish, place the remaining coconut.

6 Coat the patties in coconut evenly.

7 Now push the Temp button and rotate the dial to set the temperature at 375 degrees F.

8 Select the "Start/Pause" button to start.

9 When the unit beeps to show that it is preheated, open the lid.

10 Arrange the patties in a greased "Air Fry Basket" and insert it in the oven.

11 Serve hot.

Nutrition:

Calories 56 Total Fat 1.6 g

Saturated Fat 0.9 g

Cholesterol 35 mg

Sodium 68 mg

Total Carbs 0.7 g

Fiber 0.3 g

Sugar 0.3 g

Protein 9.3 g

108. Spicy Catfish

Difficulty: Hard

Preparation Time: 15 minutes

Cooking Time: 13 minutes

Servings: 2

Ingredients:

- tablespoons almond flour
- 1 teaspoon red chili powder
- ½ teaspoon paprika
- ½ teaspoon garlic powder
- Salt, as required
- (6-oz.) catfish fillets
- 1 tablespoon olive oil

Directions:

1 Combine the flour, paprika, garlic powder, and salt in a bowl.

2 Add the catfish fillets and coat with the mixture evenly.

3 Now, coat each fillet with oil.

4 Set the temperature at 400 degrees F.

5 When the unit beeps to show that it is preheated, open the lid.

6 Insert the fish fillets in oven.

7 Flip the fish fillets once halfway through.

8 Serve hot.

Nutrition:

Calories 340

Total Fat 23.5 g

Saturated Fat 3.7 g

Cholesterol 80 mg

Sodium 184 mg

Total Carbs 3 g

Fiber 1.5 g

Sugar 0.3 g

Protein 28.3 g

109. Seasoned Catfish

Difficulty: Hard

Preparation Time: 15 minutes

Cooking Time: 23 minutes

Servings: 4

Ingredients:

- (4-oz.) catfish fillets
- tablespoons Italian seasoning
- Salt and ground black pepper, as required
- 1 tablespoon olive oil
- 1 tablespoon fresh parsley, chopped

Directions:

1 Rub the fish fillets with seasoning, salt, and black pepper generously and then coat with oil.

2 Push the Temp button and rotate the dial to set the temperature at 400 degrees F.

3 When the unit beeps to show that it is preheated, open the lid.

4 Arrange the fish fillets in a greased "Air Fry Basket" and insert it in the oven.

5 Flip the fish fillets once halfway through.

6 Serve hot with the garnishing of parsley.

Nutrition:

Calories 205

Total Fat 14.2 g

Saturated Fat 2.4 g

Cholesterol 58 mg

Sodium 102 mg

Total Carbs 0.8 g

Fiber 0 g

Sugar 0.6 g

Protein 17.7 g

110. Crispy Catfish

Difficulty: Hard

Preparation Time: 15 minutes

Cooking Time: 15 minutes

Servings: 5

Ingredients:

- (6-oz.) catfish fillets
- 1 cup milk
- teaspoons fresh lemon juice
- ½ cup yellow mustard
- ½ cup cornmeal
- ¼ cup all-purpose flour
- tablespoons dried parsley flakes
- ¼ teaspoon red chili powder
- ¼ teaspoon cayenne pepper
- ¼ teaspoon onion powder
- ¼ teaspoon garlic powder
- Salt and ground black pepper, as required
- Olive oil cooking spray

Directions:

1. In a large bowl, place the catfish, milk, and lemon juice and refrigerate for about 15 minutes.
2. In a shallow bowl, add the mustard.
3. In another bowl, mix the cornmeal, flour, parsley flakes, and spices.
4. Remove the catfish fillets from the milk mixture, and with paper towels, pat them dry.
5. Coat each fish fillet with mustard and then roll into cornmeal mixture.
6. Then, spray each fillet with the cooking spray.
7. When the unit beeps to show that it is preheated, open the lid.
8. Assemble the catfish fillets in a "Air Fry Basket" in the oven
9. After 10 minutes of cooking, flip the fillets and spray with the cooking spray.
10. Serve hot.

Nutrition:

Calories 340

Total Fat 15.5 g

Saturated Fat 3.1 g

Cholesterol 84 mg

Sodium 435 mg

Total Carbs 18.3 g

Fiber 2 g

Sugar 2.7 g

Protein 30.9 g

111. Cornmeal Coated Catfish

Difficulty: Hard

Preparation Time: 15 minutes

Cooking Time: 14 minutes

Servings: 4

Ingredients:

- tablespoons cornmeal
- teaspoons Cajun seasoning

- ½ teaspoon paprika
- ½ teaspoon garlic powder
- Salt, as required
- (6-oz.) catfish fillets
- 1 tablespoon olive oil

Directions:

1. In a bowl, mix the cornmeal, Cajun seasoning, paprika, garlic powder, and salt.
2. Add the catfish fillets and coat with the mixture.
3. Now, coat each fillet with oil.
4. When the unit beeps to show that it is preheated, open the lid.
5. Arrange the catfish fillets in a greased "Air Fry Basket" and insert them in the oven.
6. After 10 minutes of cooking, flip the fillets and spray with the cooking spray.
7. Serve hot

Nutrition:

Calories 161

Total Fat 10.1 g

Saturated Fat 1.7 g

Cholesterol 40 mg

Sodium 110 mg

Total Carbs 3.3 g

Fiber 0.4 g

Sugar 0.1 g

Protein 13.7 g

112. Breaded Flounder

Difficulty: Hard

Preparation Time: 15 minutes

Cooking Time: 12 minutes

Servings: 3

Ingredients:

- 1 egg
- 1 cup dry breadcrumbs
- ¼ cup vegetable oil
- (6-oz.) flounder fillets
- 1 lemon, sliced

Directions:

1. Beat the egg in a bowl.
2. Put in the breadcrumbs and oil in a bowl and mix until a crumbly mixture is formed.
3. Dip flounder fillets into the beaten egg and then coat with the breadcrumb mixture.
4. When the unit beeps to show that it is preheated, open the lid.
5. Arrange the flounder fillets in a greased "Air Fry Basket" and insert it in the oven.
6. Set off with the lemon slices and serve hot.

Nutrition:

Calories 524 Total Fat 24.2 g

Saturated Fat 5.1 g Cholesterol 170 mg

Sodium 463 mg Total Carbs 26.5 g

Fiber 1.5 g Sugar 2.5 g

Protein 47.8g

CHAPTER 7:

Vegetables

113. Mushroom and Feta Frittata

Difficulty: Very Easy

Preparation Time: 5 minutes

Cooking Time: 30 minutes

Servings: 4

Ingredients:

- cups button mushrooms
- red onion
- tablespoons olive oil
- tablespoons feta cheese, crumbled
- Pinch of salt
- eggs
- Cooking spray

Directions:

1 Add olive oil to pan and sauté mushrooms over medium heat until tender. Remove from heat and pan so that they can cool. Preheat your air fryer to 330 degree F.

2 Add cracked eggs into a bowl, and whisk them, adding a pinch of salt. Coat an 8-inch heat resistant baking dish with cooking spray. Add the eggs into the baking dish, then onion and mushroom mixture, and then add feta cheese.

3 Place the baking dish into air fryer for 30-minutes and serve warm.

Nutrition:

Calories: 246 kcal/Cal

Total Fat: 12.3 g

Carbohydrates: 9.2 g

Protein: 10.3 g

114. Cauliflower pizza crust

Difficulty: Very Easy

Preparation Time: 26 minutes

Cooking Time: 20 minutes

Servings: 2

Ingredients:

- 1 (12-oz.) Steamer bag cauliflower
- 1 large egg.
- ½ cup shredded sharp cheddar cheese.
- tbsp. Blanched finely ground almond flour
- 1 tsp. Italian blend seasoning

Directions:

1. Cook the cauliflower according to the directions on the package. Take it out of the bag and place it on a cheesecloth or paper towel to remove excess water. Place the cauliflower in a large bowl.

2. Cut a piece of parchment to fit in the fryer basket. Press cauliflower into a 6-inch round circle. Place in the fryer basket. Set the temperature to 360 ° F and set the

timer for 11 minutes. After 7 minutes, turn the pizza dough over.

3. Add your favorite garnish to the pizza. Place back in the fryer basket and cook an additional 4 minutes or until fully cooked and golden. Serve immediately.

Nutrition:

Calories: 230 kcal/Cal Protein: 14.9 g

Fiber: 4.7 g Fat: 14.2 g Carbohydrates: 10.0 g

115. Olives and artichokes

Difficulty: Very Easy

Preparation Time: 20 minutes

Cooking Time: 15 minutes

Servings: 4

Ingredients:

- oz. canned artichoke hearts, drained
- ½ cup tomato sauce
- cups black olives, pitted
- garlic cloves; minced
- 1 tbsp. Olive oil
- 1 tsp. Garlic powder

Dircctions:

1 In a pan that fits your air fryer, mix the olives with the artichokes and the other ingredients, toss,

2 put the pan in the fryer and cook at 350°f for 15 minutes

Divide the mix between plates and serve.

Nutrition:

Calories: 180 kcal/Cal

Fat: 4 g Fiber: 3 g

Carbohydrates: 5 g Protein: 6 g

116. Lemon asparagus

Difficulty: Very Easy

Preparation Time: 17 minutes

Cooking Time: 12 minutes

Servings: 4

Ingredients:

- 1 lb. Asparagus, trimmed
- garlic cloves; minced
- tbsp. Parmesan, grated
- tbsp. Olive oil
- Juice of 1 lemon
- A pinch of salt and black pepper

Directions:

1 Take a bowl and mix the asparagus with the rest of the ingredients and toss.

2 Put the asparagus in your air fryer's basket and cook at 390°F for 12 minutes. Divide between plates and serve!

Nutrition:

Calories: 175 kcal/Cal Fat: 5 g

Fiber: 2 g Carbohydrates: 4 g Protein: 8 g

117. Savory cabbage and tomatoes

Difficulty: Very Easy

Preparation Time: 20 minutes

Cooking Time: 15 minutes

Servings: 4

Ingredients:

- Spring onions; chopped.
- 1 savoy cabbage, shredded

- 1 tbsp. Parsley; chopped.
- tbsp. Tomato sauce
- Salt and black pepper to taste.

Directions:

1. In a pan that fits your air fryer, mix the cabbage the rest of the ingredients except the parsley, toss, put the pan in the fryer and cook at 360°f for 15 minutes
2. Divide between plates and serve with parsley sprinkled on top.

Nutrition:

Calories: 163 kcal/Cal

Fat: 4 g Fiber: 3 g

Carbohydrates: 6 g

Protein: 7 g

118. Pecan brownies

Difficulty: Very Easy

Preparation Time: 30 minutes

Cooking Time: 20 minutes

Servings: 6

Ingredients:

- ¼ cup chopped pecans
- ¼ cup low carb
- Sugar: -free chocolate chips.
- ¼ cup unsalted butter; softened.
- 1 large egg.
- ½ cup blanched finely ground almond flour.
- ½ cup powdered erythritol
- tbsp. Unsweetened cocoa powder
- ½ tsp. Baking powder.

Directions:

1. Take a bowl, mix almond flour, erythritol, cocoa powder and baking powder. Stir in butter and egg.
2. Adjust the temperature to 300°F and set the timer for 20 minutes. When fully cooked a toothpick inserted in center will come out clean. Allow 20 minutes to fully cool and firm up.

Nutrition:

Calories: 215 kcal/Cal

Protein: 4.2 g

Fiber: 2.8 g

Fat: 18.9 g

Carbohydrates: 21.8 g

119. Cheesy endives

Difficulty: Very Easy

Preparation Time: 20 minutes

Cooking Time: 15 minutes

Servings: 4

Ingredients:

- endives, trimmed
- ¼ cup goat cheese, crumbled
- 1 tbsp. Lemon juice
- Tbsp. Chives; chopped.
- tbsp. Olive oil
- 1 tsp. Lemon zest, grated
- A pinch of salt and black pepper

Directions:

1. Take a bowl and mix the endives with the other ingredients except the cheese and chives and toss well.

2 Put the endives in your air fryer's basket and cook at 380°F for 15 minutes

3 Divide the corn between plates.

4 Serve with cheese and chives sprinkled on top.

Nutrition:

Calories: 140 kcal/Cal

Fat: 4 g

Fiber: 3 g

Carbohydrates: 5 g

Protein: 7 g

120. Cauliflower steak

Difficulty: Easy

Preparation Time: 12 minutes

Cooking Time: 7 minutes

Servings: 4

Ingredients:

- 1 medium head cauliflower
- ¼ cup blue cheese crumbles
- ¼ cup hot sauce
- ¼ cup full-fat ranch dressing
- 1 tbsp. Salted butter; melted.

Directions:

1 Remove cauliflower leaves. Slice the head in ½-inch-thick slices.

2 In a small bowl, mix hot sauce and butter. Brush the mixture over the cauliflower.

3 Place each cauliflower steak into the air fryer, working in batches if necessary. Adjust the temperature to 400°F and set the timer for 7 minutes

4 When cooked, edges will begin turning dark and caramelized. To serve, sprinkle steaks with crumbled blue cheese. Drizzle with ranch dressing.

Nutrition:

Calories: 122 kcal/Cal Protein: 4.9 g

Fiber: 3.0 g Fat: 8.4 g Carbohydrates: 7.7 g

121. Parmesan Broccoli and Asparagus

Difficulty: Easy

Preparation Time: 20 minutes

Cooking Time: 15 minutes

Servings: 4

Ingredients:

- ½ lb. asparagus, trimmed
- 1 broccoli head, florets separated
- Juice of 1 lime
- tbsp. parmesan, grated
- tbsp. olive oil
- Salt and black pepper to taste.

Directions:

1 Take a bowl and mix the asparagus with the broccoli and all the other ingredients except the parmesan, toss, transfer to your air fryer's basket and cook at 400°F for 15 minutes

2 Divide between plates, sprinkle the parmesan on top and serve.

Nutrition:

Calories: 172 kcal/Cal Fat: 5 g

Fiber: 2 g Carbohydrates: 4 g

Protein: 9 g

122. Air Fryer Crunchy Cauliflower

Difficulty: Easy

Preparation Time: 20 minutes

Cooking Time: 15 minutes

Servings: 5

Ingredients:

- oz. cauliflower
- 1 tbsp. potato starch
- 1 tsp. olive oil
- Salt & pepper to taste

Directions:

1. Set the air fryer toaster oven to 400°F and preheat it for 3 minutes. Slice cauliflower into equal pieces and if you are using potato starch then toss with the florets into bowl.
2. Add some olive oil and mix to coat.
3. Use olive oil cooking spray for spraying the inside of air fryer toaster oven basket then add cauliflower.
4. Cook for eight minutes then shake the basket and cook for another 5 minutes depending on your desired level of crisp. Sprinkle roasted cauliflower with fresh parsley, kosher salt, and your seasonings or sauce of your choice.

Nutrition:

Calories: 36 kcal/Cal

Fat: 1 g

Protein: 1 g

Carbs: 5 g

Fiber: 2 g

123. Air Fryer Veg Buffalo Cauliflower

Difficulty: Easy

Preparation Time: 20 minutes

Cooking Time: 15 minutes

Servings: 3

Ingredients:

- 1 medium head cauliflower
- tsp. avocado oil
- tbsp. red hot sauce
- tbsp. nutritional yeast
- 1 1/2 tsp. maple syrup
- 1/4 tsp. sea salt
- 1 tbsp. cornstarch or arrowroot starch

Directions:

1 Set your air fryer toaster oven to 360°F. Place all the ingredients to bowl except cauliflower. Mix them to combine.

2 Put the cauliflower and mix to coat equally. Put half of your cauliflower to air fryer and cook for 15 minutes but keep shaking them until your get desired consistency.

3 Do the same for the cauliflower which is left except lower cooking time to 10 minutes.

4 Keep the cauliflower tightly sealed in refrigerator for 3-4 days. For heating again add back to air fryer for 1-2 minutes until crispness.

Nutrition:

Calories: 248 kcal/Cal Fat: 20g

Protein: 4g Carbs: 13g

Fiber: 2g

124. Air Fryer Asparagus

Difficulty: Easy

Preparation Time: 5 minutes

Cooking Time: 13 minutes

Servings: 2

Ingredients:

- Nutritional yeast
- Olive oil nonstick spray
- One bunch of asparagus

Directions:

1 Wash asparagus and then trim off thick, woody ends.

2 Spray asparagus with olive oil spray and sprinkle with yeast.

3 Add the asparagus to air fryer rack/basket in a singular layer. Set temperature to 360°F and set time to 8 minutes. Select START/STOP to begin.

Nutrition:

Calories: 17 kcal/Cal

Total Fat: 8 g

Total Carbs: 2 g

Protein: 9 g

125. Almond Flour Battered and Crisped Onion Rings

Difficulty: Medium

Preparation Time: 5 minutes

Cooking Time: 20 minutes

Servings: 3

Ingredients:

- ½ cup almond flour
- ¾ cup coconut milk
- 1 big white onion, sliced into rings
- 1 egg, beaten
- 1 tablespoon baking powder
- 1 tablespoon smoked paprika
- Salt and pepper to taste

Directions:

1 Preheat the air fryer Oven for 5 minutes.

2 In a mixing bowl, mix the almond flour, baking powder, smoked paprika, salt and pepper.

3 In another bowl, combine the eggs and coconut milk.

4 Soak the onion slices into the egg mixture.

5 Dredge the onion slices in the almond flour mixture.

6 Pour into the Oven rack/basket. Set temperature to 325°F and set time to 15 minutes. Select START/STOP to begin. Shake the fryer basket for even cooking.

Nutrition:

Calories: 217 kcal/Cal Total Fat: 17 g

Total Carbs: 2 g Fiber: 6 g Protein: 5 g

126. Divided Balsamic Mustard Greens

Difficulty: Medium

Preparation Time: 17 minutes;

Cooking Time: 15 minutes

Servings: 4

Ingredients:

- mustard greens - 1 bunch, trimmed
- olive oil - 2 tablespoons

- chicken stock - ½ cup
- tomato puree - 2 tablespoons
- garlic cloves - 3, minced
- Salt and black pepper to taste
- balsamic vinegar - 1 tablespoon

Directions:

1 Mix all of the ingredients in a pan that fits right into your air fryer and toss well.
2 Move the pan to the fryer and cook at a temperature of 260 o F for 12 minutes.
3 Divide all of it into different plates, serve your meal, and enjoy!

Nutrition:

Calories 151, Fat 2, Fiber 4,

Carbs 14, Protein 4

127. Butter Endives Recipe

Difficulty: Medium

Preparation Time: 15 minutes;

Cooking Time: 15 minutes

Servings: 4

Ingredients:

- Endives - 4, trimmed and halved
- Salt and black pepper to taste
- lime juice - 1 tablespoon
- Butter - 1 tablespoon, melted

Directions:

1 Place the endives in your air fryer, then add the salt and pepper to taste, lemon juice, and butter.
2 Cook at a temperature of 360 o F for 10 minutes.
3 Cut into different plates and serve right away.

Nutrition:

Calories 100, Fat 3,

Fiber 4, Carbs 8, Protein 4

128. Endives with Bacon Mix

Difficulty: Medium

Preparation Time: 15 minutes;

Cooking Time: 15 minutes

Servings: 4

Ingredients:

- Endives - 4, trimmed and halved
- Salt and black pepper to taste
- olive oil - 1 tablespoon
- bacon - 2 tablespoons, cooked and crumbled
- nutmeg - ½ teaspoon, ground

Directions:

1 Place the endives in your air fryer's basket, then add the salt and pepper to taste as well as oil and nutmeg; ensure to toss gently.
2 Cook at a temperature of 360 o F for 10 minutes.
3 Cut the endives into different plates, then sprinkle the bacon as toppings, and serve.

Nutrition:

Calories 151,

Fat 6,

Fiber 8,

Carbs 14,

Protein 6

129. Sweet Beets Salad

Difficulty: Medium

Preparation Time: 20 Minutes

Cooking Time: 15 minutes

Servings: 4

Ingredients:

- Beets; peeled and quartered-1 ½-pound
- Brown sugar-2 tbsps.
- Scallions; chopped-2
- Cider vinegar-2 tbsps.
- Orange juice-1/2 cup
- Arugula-2 cups
- Mustard-2 tsps.
- Olive oil- a drizzle
- Orange zest; grated-2 tsps.

Directions:

4 Season the beets with orange juice and oil in a bowl.
5 Spread the beets in the air fryer basket and seal the fryer.
6 Cook the beet for 10 minutes at 3500 F on Air fryer mode.
7 Place these cooked beets in a bowl then toss in orange zest, arugula, and scallions.
8 Whisk mustard, vinegar, and sugar in a different bowl.
9 Add this mixture to the beets and mix well.
10 Enjoy.

Nutrition:

Calories 151, Fat 2,

Fiber 4, Carbs 14,

Protein 4

130. Cheesy Cauliflower Fritters

Difficulty: Medium

Preparation Time: 5 minutes

Cooking Time: 14 minutes

Servings: 8

Ingredients:

- ½ C. chopped parsley
- 1 C. Italian breadcrumbs
- 1/3 C. shredded mozzarella cheese
- 1/3 C. shredded sharp cheddar cheese
- 1 egg
- minced garlic cloves
- chopped scallions
- 1 head of cauliflower

Directions:

1 Cut cauliflower up into florets. Wash well and pat dry. Place into a food processor and pulse 20-30 seconds till it looks like rice.
2 Place cauliflower rice in a bowl and mix with pepper, salt, egg, cheeses, breadcrumbs, garlic, and scallions.
3 With hands, form 15 patties of the mixture. Add more breadcrumbs if needed.
4 With olive oil, spritz patties, and place into your air fryer in a single layer.
5 Cook 14 minutes at 390 degrees, flipping after 7 minutes.

Nutrition:

Calories: 209

Fat: 17g

Protein: 6g

Sugar: 0.5g

131. Avocado Fries

Difficulty: Medium

Preparation Time: 5 minutes

Cooking Time: 5 minutes

Servings: 6

Ingredients:

- 1 avocado
- ½ tsp. salt
- ½ C. panko breadcrumbs
- Bean liquid (aquafaba) from a 15-ounce can of white or garbanzo beans

Directions:

1 Peel, pit, and slice up avocado.
2 Toss salt and breadcrumbs together in a bowl. Place aquafaba into another bowl.
3 Dredge slices of avocado first in aquafaba and then in panko, making sure you get an even coating.
4 Place coated avocado slices into a single layer in the air fryer.
5 Cook 5 minutes at 390 degrees, shaking at 5 minutes. Serve with your favorite dipping sauce!

Nutrition:

Calories: 102 Fat: 22gProtein: 9g Sugar: 1g

132. Zucchini Parmesan Chips

Difficulty: Hard

Preparation Time: 5 minutes

Cooking Time: 8 minutes

Servings: 10

Ingredients:

- ½ tsp. paprika
- ½ C. grated parmesan cheese
- ½ C. Italian breadcrumbs
- 1 lightly beaten egg
- thinly sliced zucchinis

Directions:

1 Use a very sharp knife or mandolin slicer to slice zucchini as thinly as you can. Pat off extra moisture.
2 Beat egg with a pinch of pepper and salt and a bit of water.
3 Combine paprika, cheese, and breadcrumbs in a bowl.
4 Dip slices of zucchini into the egg mixture and then into breadcrumb mixture. Press gently to coat.
5 With olive oil cooking spray, mist coated zucchini slices. Place into your air fryer in a single layer.
6 Cook 8 minutes at 350 degrees.
7 Sprinkle with salt and serve with salsa.

Nutrition:

Calories: 211 Fat: 16g Protein: 8g Sugar: 0g

133. Crispy Roasted Broccoli

Difficulty: Hard

Preparation Time: 45 minutes

Cooking Time: 15 minutes

Servings: 2

Ingredients:

- ¼ tsp. Masala
- ½ tsp. red chili powder
- ½ tsp. salt
- ¼ tsp. turmeric powder
- 1 tbsp. chickpea flour
- tbsp. yogurt
- 1-pound broccoli

Directions:

1 Cut broccoli up into florets. Soak in a bowl of water with 2 teaspoons of salt for at least half an hour to remove impurities.
2 Take out broccoli florets from water and let drain. Wipe down thoroughly.
3 Mix all other ingredients together to create a marinade.
4 Toss broccoli florets in the marinade. Cover and chill 15-30 minutes.
5 Preheat air fryer to 390 degrees. Place marinated broccoli florets into the fryer. Cook 10 minutes.
6 6 minutes into cooking shake the basket. Florets will be crispy when done.

Nutrition:

Calories: 96 Fat: 1.3g Protein: 7g Sugar: 4.5g

134. Crispy Jalapeno Coins

Difficulty: Hard

Preparation Time: 10 minutes

Cooking Time: 10 minutes

Servings: 8 to 10

Ingredients:

- 1 egg
- 2-3 tbsp. coconut flour
- 1 sliced and seeded jalapeno
- Pinch of garlic powder
- Pinch of onion powder
- Bit of Cajun seasoning (optional)
- Pinch of pepper and salt

Directions:

1 Ensure your air fryer is preheated to 400 degrees.
2 Mix together all dry ingredients.
3 Pat jalapeno slices dry. Dip coins into egg wash and then into dry mixture. Toss to coat thoroughly.
4 Add coated jalapeno slices to air fryer in a singular layer. Spray with olive oil.
5 Cook just till crispy.

Nutrition:

Calories: 128

Fat: 8g

Protein: 7g

Sugar: 0g

135. Buffalo Cauliflower

Difficulty: Hard

Preparation Time: 15 minutes

Cooking Time: 14 to 17 minutes

Servings: 6 to 8

Ingredients:

- Cauliflower:
- 1 C. panko breadcrumbs
- 1 tsp. salt
- C. cauliflower florets
- Buffalo Coating:
- ¼ C. Vegan Buffalo sauce
- ¼ C. melted vegan butter

Directions:

1 Melt butter in microwave and whisk in buffalo sauce.
2 Dip each cauliflower floret into buffalo mixture, ensuring it gets coated well. Hold over a bowl till floret is done dripping.
3 Mix breadcrumbs with salt.

4 Dredge dipped florets into breadcrumbs and place into air fryer.
5 Cook 14-17 minutes at 350 degrees. When slightly browned, they are ready to eat!
6 Serve with your favorite keto dipping sauce!

Nutrition:

Calories: 194 Fat: 17g Protein: 10g Sugar: 3g

136. Jicama Fries

Difficulty: Hard

Preparation Time: 10 minutes

Cooking Time: 20 minutes

Servings: 8

Ingredients:

- 1 tbsp. dried thyme
- ¾ C. arrowroot flour
- ½ large Jicama
- eggs

Directions:

1 Sliced jicama into fries.
2 Whisk eggs together and pour over fries. Toss to coat.
3 Mix a pinch of salt, thyme, and arrowroot flour together. Toss egg-coated jicama into dry mixture, tossing to coat well.
4 Spray air fryer basket with olive oil and add fries. Cook 20 minutes on CHIPS setting. Toss halfway into the cooking process.

Nutrition:

Calories: 211 Fat: 19g

Protein: 9g Sugar: 1g

137. Air Fryer Brussels Sprouts

Difficulty: Hard

Preparation Time: 5 minutes

Cooking Time: 10 minutes

Servings: 5

Ingredients:

- ¼ tsp. salt
- 1 tbsp. balsamic vinegar
- 1 tbsp. olive oil
- C. Brussels sprouts

Directions:

1 Cut Brussels sprouts in half lengthwise. Toss with salt, vinegar, and olive oil till coated thoroughly.
2 Add coated sprouts to air fryer, cooking 8-10 minutes at 400 degrees. Shake after 5 minutes of cooking.
3 Brussels sprouts are ready to devour when brown and crisp!

Nutrition:

Calories: 118 Fat: 9g

Protein: 11g Sugar: 1g

138. Spaghetti Squash Tots

Difficulty: Hard

Preparation Time: 5 minutes

Cooking Time: 15 minutes

Servings: 8 to 10

Ingredients:

- ¼ tsp. pepper
- ½ tsp. salt
- 1 thinly sliced scallion
- 1 spaghetti squash

Directions:

1 Wash and cut the squash in half lengthwise. Scrape out the seeds.
2 With a fork, remove spaghetti meat by strands and throw out skins.
3 In a clean towel, toss in squash and wring out as much moisture as possible. Place in a bowl and with a knife slice through meat a few times to cut up smaller.
4 Add pepper, salt, and scallions to squash and mix well.
5 Create "tot" shapes with your hands and place in air fryer. Spray with olive oil.
6 Cook 15 minutes at 350 degrees until golden and crispy!

Nutrition:

Calories: 231

Fat: 18g

Protein: 5g Sugar: 0g

139. Cinnamon Butternut Squash Fries

Difficulty: Very Hard

Preparation Time: 10 minutes

Cooking Time: 10 minutes

Servings: 2

Ingredients:

- 1 pinch of salt
- 1 tbsp. powdered unprocessed sugar
- ½ tsp. nutmeg
- tsp. cinnamon
- 1 tbsp. coconut oil
- ounces pre-cut butternut squash fries

Directions:

1 In a plastic bag, pour in all ingredients. Coat fries with other components till coated and sugar is dissolved.
2 Spread coated fries into a single layer in the air fryer. Cook 10 minutes at 390 degrees until crispy.

Nutrition:

Calories: 175

Fat: 8g

Protein: 1g

Sugar: 5g

140. Carrot & Zucchini Muffins

Difficulty: Very Hard

Preparation Time: 5 minutes

Cooking Time: 14 minutes

Servings: 4

Ingredients:

- tablespoons butter, melted
- ¼ cup carrots, shredded
- ½ cup zucchini, shredded
- 1 ½ cups almond flour
- 1 tablespoon liquid Stevia
- teaspoons baking powder
- Pinch of salt
- eggs
- 1 tablespoon yogurt
- 1 cup milk

Directions:

1 Preheat your air fryer to 350 degree Fahrenheit.
2 Beat the eggs, yogurt, milk, salt, pepper, baking soda, and Stevia.
3 Whisk in the flour gradually.

4 Add zucchini and carrots.
5 Grease muffin tins with butter and pour muffin batter into containers. Cook for 14-minutes and serve.

Nutrition:

Calories: 224,

Total Fats: 12.3g,

Carbs: 11.2g,

Protein: 14.2g

141. Curried Cauliflower Florets

Difficulty: Very Hard

Preparation Time: 5 minutes

Cooking Time: 10 minutes

Servings: 4

Ingredients:

- 1/4 cup sultanas or golden raisins
- ¼ teaspoon salt
- 1 tablespoon curry powder
- 1 head cauliflower, broken into small florets
- ¼ cup pine nuts
- ½ cup olive oil

Directions:

1. In a cup of boiling water, soak your sultanas to plump. Preheat your air fryer to 350 degree Fahrenheit.
2. Add oil and pine nuts to air fryer and toast for a minute or so.
3. In a bowl toss the cauliflower and curry powder as well as salt, then add the mix to air fryer mixing well.
4. Cook for 10-minutes. Drain the sultanas, toss with cauliflower, and serve.

Nutrition:

Calories: 275,

Total Fat: 11.3g,

Carbs: 8.6g,

Protein: 9.5g

142. Crispy Rye Bread Snacks with Guacamole and Anchovies

Difficulty: Very Hard

Preparation Time: 10 minutes

Cooking Time: 10 minutes

Servings: 4

Ingredients:

- slices of rye bread
- Guacamole
- Anchovies in oil

Directions:

1 Cut each slice of bread into 3 strips of bread.
2 Place in the basket of the air fryer, without piling up, and we go in batches giving it the touch you want to give it. You can select 3500F, 10 minutes.
3 When you have all the crusty rye bread strips, put a layer of guacamole on top, whether homemade or commercial.
4 In each bread, place 2 anchovies on the guacamole.

Nutrition:

Calories: 180 Fat: 11.6g

Carbohydrates: 16g Protein: 6.2g

Sugar: 0g Cholesterol: 19.6mg

143. Oat and Chia Porridge

Difficulty: Very Hard

Preparation Time: 5 minutes

Cooking Time: 5 minutes

Servings: 4

Ingredients:

- tablespoons peanut butter
- teaspoons liquid Stevia
- 1 tablespoon butter, melted
- cups milk
- cups oats
- 1 cup chia seeds

Directions:

1. Preheat your air fryer to 390 degree Fahrenheit.
2. Whisk the peanut butter, butter, milk and Stevia in a bowl.
3. Stir in the oats and chia seeds.
4. Pour the mixture into an oven-proof bowl and place in the air fryer and cook for 5-minutes.

Nutrition:

Calories: 228, Total Fats: 11.4g,

Carbs: 10.2g, Protein: 14.5g

144. Feta & Mushroom Frittata

Difficulty: Very Hard

Preparation Time: 15 minutes

Cooking Time: 30 minutes

Servings: 4

Ingredients:

- 1 red onion, thinly sliced
- cups button mushrooms, thinly sliced
- Salt to taste
- tablespoons feta cheese, crumbled
- medium eggs
- Non-stick cooking spray
- tablespoons olive oil

Directions:

1. Saute the onion and mushrooms in olive oil over medium heat until the vegetables are tender.
2. Remove the vegetables from pan and drain on a paper towel-lined plate.
3. In a mixing bowl, whisk eggs and salt. Coat all sides of baking dish with cooking spray.
4. Preheat your air fryer to 325 degree Fahrenheit. Pour the beaten eggs into prepared baking dish and scatter the sautéed vegetables and crumble feta on top. Bake in the air fryer for 30-minutes. Allow to cool slightly and serve!

Nutrition:

Calories: 226, Total Fat: 9.3g,

Carbs: 8.7g, Protein: 12.6g

145. Butter Glazed Carrots

Difficulty: Very Hard

Preparation Time: 20 Minutes

Cooking Time: 15 minutes

Servings: 4

Ingredients:

- Baby carrots-2 cups
- Brown sugar-1 tbsps.
- Butter; melted-1/2 tbsps.
- Salt and black pepper- a pinch

Directions:

1 Take a baking dish suitable to fit in your air fryer. Toss carrots with sugar, butter, salt and black peppers in that baking dish.

2 Place this dish in the air fryer basket and seal the fryer. Cook the carrots for 10 minutes at 3500 F on Air fryer mode. Enjoy.

Nutrition:

Calories 151,

Fat 2,

Fiber 4,

Carbs 14,

Protein 4

CHAPTER 8:

Side Dishes

146. Bacon Cheddar Chicken Fingers

Difficulty: Very Easy

Preparation Time: 8 minutes

Cooking Time: 12 minutes

Servings: 8

Ingredients:

- For the chicken fingers:
- 1 lb. chicken tenders, about 8 pieces
- cooking spray (canola oil)
- cheddar cheese - 1 cup, shredded
- Two eggs, large
- 1/3 cup bacon bits
- tbsp. water
- For the breading:
- 1 tsp. of onion powder
- panko bread crumbs - 2 cups
- black pepper - 1 tsp., freshly ground
- Paprika - 2 tbsp.
- Garlic powder - 1 tsp.
- Salt - 2 tsp.

Directions:

1. Set the air fryer to the temperature of 360°F.
2. In a glass dish, whip the water and eggs until combined.
3. Use a zip lock bag, shake the garlic powder, salt, breadcrumbs, cayenne, onion powder, and pepper together.
4. Immerse the chicken into the eggs and shake in the zip lock bag until fully covered.
5. Dip again in the mixture of egg and back into the seasonings until a thick coating is present.
6. Remove the tenders from the bag and set in the frying pan in the basket. Do them in batches if you need to not over pack the pan.
7. Apply the canola oil spray to the top of the tenders and heat for 6 minutes.
8. Flip the tenders to the other side. Steam for another 4 minutes.
9. Blend the bacon bits and shredded cheese in a dish.
10. Evenly dust the bacon and cheese onto the hot tenders and fry for 2 more minutes.

11 Remove and serve while hot.

Nutrition:

Calories 320,

Fat 25,

Fiber 17,

Carbs 37,

Protein 40

147. Battered Cod

Difficulty: Very Easy

Preparation Time: 16 minutes

Cooking Time: 14 minutes

Servings: 2

Ingredients:

- Cod - 20 oz.
- Salt - 1/4 tsp.
- All-purpose flour - 8 oz.
- Parsley seasoning - 1 tbsp.
- Cornstarch - 3 tsp.
- Garlic powder - 1/2 tsp.
- Two eggs, preferably large
- Onion powder - 1/2 tsp.

Directions:

1 Whip the eggs in a glass dish until smooth and set to the side.

2 In a separate dish, blend the cornstarch, salt, almond flour, garlic powder, parsley, and onion powder, whisking to remove any lumpiness.

3 Immerse the pieces of cods into the egg and then into the spiced flour, covering completely.

4 Transfer to the fryer basket in a single layer.

5 Heat the fish for 7 minutes at a temperature of 350°F. Turn the cod over and steam for an additional 7 minutes.

Nutrition:

Calories 254,

Fat 4,

Fiber 10,

Carbs 17,

Protein 12

148. Beef Kabobs

Difficulty: Very Easy

Preparation Time: 10 minutes

Cooking Time: 12 minutes

Servings: 3

Ingredients:

- Low-fat sour cream - 1/3 cup
- One bell pepper
- 4 oz. Of beef chuck ribs, boneless
- Soy sauce - 2 tbsp.
- 6-inch skewers - 8
- Pepper - 1/4 tsp.
- Medium onion - 1/2

Directions:

1 Slice the ribs into sections about 1-inch wide
2 In a lidded tub, combine the soy sauce, ribs, and sour cream, making sure the meat is fully covered.
3 Refrigerate for half an hour, at least, if not overnight. Immerse the wooden skewers for approximately 10 minutes in water.
4 Set the temperature of the air fryer oven to 400°F.
5 Slice the onion and bell pepper in 1-inch sections.
6 Remove the meat from the marinade, draining well. Layer the onions, beef, and bell peppers on the skewers and dust with pepper.
7 Heat for 10 minutes, ensuring you spin the skewers 5 minutes into cooking time. Serve while hot and enjoy.

Nutrition:

Calories 312, Fat 10, Fiber 8, Carbs 29, Protein 30

149. Cheese Dogs

Difficulty: Very Easy

Preparation Time: 3 minutes

Cooking Time: 10 minutes

Servings: 7

Ingredients:

- hotdogs
- 1/4 cup your choice of cheese, grated
- hotdog buns

Directions:

1 Adjust the air fryer to heat at a temperature of 390°F for approximately 5 minutes.
2 Set the hot dogs in the basket and broil for 5 minutes.
3 Remove and create the hot dog with the bun and cheese as desired and move back to the basket for another 2 minutes.
4 Remove and enjoy while hot.

Nutrition:

Calories 200,

Fat 5,

Fiber 10,

Carbs 17,

Protein 18

150. Cheeseburger Patties

Difficulty: Very Easy

Preparation Time: 10 minutes

Cooking Time: 13 minutes

Servings: 4

Ingredients:

- Garlic - 1/2 clove, minced
- Ground beef - 1 1/3 cup
- Onion - 4 oz., diced
- Worcestershire sauce - 2 tbsp.
- One egg, large
- Panko breadcrumbs - 2 oz.
- Cayenne pepper - 1/8 tsp.

- Cooking spray (olive oil)
- Salt - 1/4 tsp.
- slices of cheese of your choice
- 1/8 tsp. Pepper

Directions:

1 Using a big glass dish, combine the diced onion, pepper, minced garlic, cayenne pepper, breadcrumbs, and salt until incorporated.

2 Blend the ground beef, Worcestershire sauce, and egg and integrate thoroughly by hand.

3 Form the meat into 4 individual patties and move to the air fryer basket.

4 Coat the patties with cooking spray.

5 Adjust the temperature for 375°F and heat for 8 minutes.

6 Turn the burgers over and steam for an additional 2 minutes.

7 Cover with a slice of cheese and continue cooking for approximately 3 minutes.

8 Enjoy or place on a bun with your favorite toppings.

Nutrition:

Calories 287,

Fat 6,

Fiber 12,

Carbs 11,

Protein 21

151. Chicken Cordon Bleu

Difficulty: Very Easy

Preparation Time: 15 minutes

Cooking Time: 20 minutes

Servings: 2

Ingredients:

- Pepper - 1/4 tsp.
- Chicken paillards - 4
- Salt - 1/4 tsp.
- Swiss cheese - 8 slices
- All-purpose flour - 1/2 cup
- Parmesan cheese - 2/3 cup, grated
- Panko breadcrumbs - 1 1/2 cup
- Ham - 8 slices
- Two eggs, large
- Dijon mustard - 2 tbsp.
- toothpicks
- Grapeseed oil spray

Directions:

1 On a section of baking lining, brush the Dijon mustard on each chicken paillard and sprinkle with pepper and salt

2 Layer 1 cheese, 2 slices of the ham and then the additional slice of cheese on each of the pieces of chicken.

3 Rotate the chicken beginning with the longer side to create a roll. Fasten in place with two toothpicks.

4 Whip the egg in one dish, empty the flour into a second dish and blend the

parmesan cheese and breadcrumbs into a third.

5 Immerse one chicken first in flour, secondly immerse in the egg and then roll the chicken completely in the breadcrumbs. Press the cheese and breadcrumbs into the chicken to secure and place onto a plate.

6 Repeat for the other pieces of chicken.

7 Apply the grapeseed oil spray to each section of chicken and transfer to the air fryer basket after 5 minutes.

8 Set the air fryer temperature to heat at 350°. Grill for 8 minutes and carefully turn the chicken to the other side—heat for an additional 8 minutes.

9 Remove to a serving dish and wait approximately 5 minutes before serving hot.

Nutrition:

Calories 176, Fat 22, Fiber 20,

Carbs 33, Protein 12

152. Buttered Corn

Difficulty: Easy

Preparation Time: 5 minutes

Cooking Time: 20 minutes

Servings: 2

Ingredients:

- Corn on the cob
- Salt and freshly ground black pepper, as needed
- Tablespoons butter, softened and divided

Directions:

1 Sprinkle the cobs evenly with salt and black pepper.

2 Then, rub with 1 tablespoon of butter.

3 With 1 piece of foil, wrap each cob.

4 Press "Power Button" of Air Fry Oven and turn the dial to select the "Air Fry" mode.

5 Press the Time button and again turn the dial to set the cooking time to 20 minutes.

6 Now push the Temp button and rotate the dial to set the temperature at 320 degrees F.

7 Press "Start/Pause" button to start.

8 When the unit beeps to show that it is preheated, open the lid.

9 Arrange the cobs in "Air Fry Basket" and insert in the oven.

10 Serve warm.

Nutrition:

Calories 186

Total Fat 12.2 g

Saturated Fat 7.4 g

Cholesterol 31 mg

Sodium 163 mg

Total Carbs 20.1 g

Fiber 2..5 g

Sugar 3.2g

Protein 2.9 g

153. Bread Sticks

Difficulty: Easy

Preparation Time: 15 minutes

Cooking Time: 6 minutes

Servings: 6

Ingredients:

- 1 egg 1/8 teaspoon ground cinnamon
- Salt, to taste
- bread slices
- Pinch of nutmeg pinch of ground cloves
- 1 tablespoon butter, softened
- Nonstick cooking spray
- 1 tablespoon icing sugar

Directions:

1 In a bowl, add the eggs, cinnamon, nutmeg, cloves, and salt and beat until well combined.

2 Spread the butter over both sides of the slices evenly.

3 Cut each bread slice into strips.

4 Dip bread strips into egg mixture evenly.

5 Press the "Power Button" of Air Fry Oven and turn the dial to select the "Air Fry" mode.

6 Press the Time button and again turn the dial to set the cooking time to 6 minutes.

7 Now push the Temp button and rotate the dial to set the temperature at 355 degrees F.

8 Press the "Start/Pause" button to start.

9 When the unit beeps to show that it is preheated, open the lid.

10 Arrange the breadsticks in "Air Fry Basket" and insert it in the oven.

11 After 2 minutes of cooking, spray both sides of the bread strips with cooking spray.

12 Serve immediately with the topping of icing sugar.

Nutrition:

Calories 41 Total Fat 2.8 g

Saturated Fat 1.5 g

Cholesterol 32 mg

Sodium 72 mg

Total Carbs 3 g

Fiber 0.1 g

Sugar 1.5 g

Protein 1.2 g

154. Polenta Sticks

Difficulty: Easy

Preparation Time: 15 minutes

Cooking Time: 6 minutes

Servings: 4

Ingredients:

- 1 tablespoon oil
- 2½ cups cooked polenta
- Salt, to taste
- ¼ cup Parmesan cheese

Directions:

1 Place the polenta in a lightly greased baking pan.

2 With a plastic wrap, cover, and refrigerate for about 1 hour or until set.

3 Remove from the refrigerator and cut into desired sized slices.

4 Sprinkle with salt.

5 Press the "Power Button" of Air Fry Oven and turn the dial to select the "Air Fry" mode.

6 Press the Time button and again turn the dial to set the cooking time to 6 minutes.

7 Now push the Temp button and rotate the dial to set the temperature at 350 degrees F.

8 Press the "Start/Pause" button to start.

9 When the unit beeps to show that it is preheated, open the lid.

10 Arrange the pan over the "Wire Rack" and insert it in the oven.

11 Top with cheese and serve.

Nutrition:

Calories 397 Total Fat 5.6g

Saturated Fat 1.3 g

Cholesterol 4mg

Sodium 127 mg

Total Carbs 76.2 g

Fiber 2.5 g

Sugar 1 g

Protein 9.1 g

155. Crispy Eggplant Slices

Difficulty: Easy

Preparation Time: 15 minutes

Cooking Time: 8 minutes

Servings: 4

Ingredients:

- 1 medium eggplant, shredded and cut into ½-inch round slices
- Salt, as required
- ½ cup all-purpose flour
- eggs, beaten
- 1 cup Italian-style breadcrumbs
- ¼ cup olive oil

Directions:

1 In a colander, add the eggplant slices and sprinkle with salt. Set aside for about 45 minutes.

2 With paper towels, pat dries the eggplant slices.

3 In a shallow dish, place the flour.

4 Crack the eggs in a second dish and beat well.

5 In a third dish, mix together the oil and breadcrumbs.

6 Coat each eggplant slice with flour, then dip into beaten eggs, and finally, coat with the breadcrumbs mixture.

7 Press the "Power Button" of Air Fry Oven and turn the dial to select the "Air Fry" mode.

8 Press the Time button and again turn the dial to set the cooking time to 8 minutes.

9 Now push the Temp button and rotate the dial to set the temperature at 390 degrees F.

10 Press the "Start/Pause" button to start.

11 When the unit beeps to show that it is preheated, open the lid.

12 Arrange the eggplant slices in "Air Fry Basket" and insert it in the oven.

13 Serve warm.

Nutrition:

Calories 332 Total Fat 16.6 g

Saturated Fat 2.8 g

Cholesterol 82 mg

Sodium 270 mg

Total Carbs 38.3 g

Fiber 5.7 g

Sugar 5.3 g

Protein 9.1 g

156. Simple Cauliflower Poppers

Difficulty: Easy

Preparation Time: 10 minutes

Cooking Time: 8 minutes

Servings: 4

Ingredients:

- ½ large head cauliflower, cut into bite-sized florets
- One tablespoon olive oil
- Salt and ground black pepper, as required

Directions:

1 In a large bowl, add all the ingredients and toss to coat well.

2 Press the "Power Button" of Air Fry Oven and turn the dial to select the "Air Fry" mode.

3 Press the Time button and again turn the dial to set the cooking time to 8 minutes.

4 Now push the Temp button and rotate the dial to set the temperature at 390 degrees F.

5 Press the "Start/Pause" button to start.

6 When the unit beeps to show that it is preheated, open the lid.

7 Arrange the cauliflower florets in "Air Fry Basket" and insert it in the oven.

8 Toss the cauliflower florets once halfway through.

9 Serve warm.

Nutrition:

Calories 38

Total Fat 23.5 g

Saturated Fat 0.5 g

Cholesterol 0 mg

Sodium 49 mg

Total Carbs 1.8 g

Fiber 0.8 g

Sugar 0.8 g

Protein 0.7 g

157. Crispy Cauliflower Poppers

Difficulty: Easy

Preparation Time: 10 minutes

Cooking Time: 20 minutes

Servings: 4

Ingredients:

- 1 egg white
- 1½ tablespoons ketchup
- 1 tablespoon hot sauce
- 1/3 cup panko breadcrumbs
- cups cauliflower florets

Directions:

1 In an open bowl, mix together the egg white, ketchup and hot sauce.

2 In another bowl, place the breadcrumbs.

3 Dip the cauliflower florets in ketchup mixture and then coat with the breadcrumbs.

4 Press the "Power Button" of Air Fry Oven and turn the dial to select the "Air Fry" mode.

5 Press the Time button and again turn the dial to set the cooking time to 20 minutes.

6 Now push the Temp button and rotate the dial to set the temperature at 320 degrees F.

7 Press the "Start/Pause" button to start.

8 When the unit beeps to show that it is preheated, open the lid.

9 Arrange the cauliflower florets in "Air Fry Basket" and insert it in the oven.

10 Toss the cauliflower florets once halfway through.

11 Serve warm.

Nutrition:

Calories 55

Total Fat 0.7 g

Saturated Fat 0.3g

Cholesterol 0 mg

Sodium 181 mg

Total Carbs 5.6 g

Fiber 1.3 g

Sugar 2.6 g

Protein 2.3 g

158. Broccoli Poppers

Difficulty: Easy

Preparation Time: 15 minutes

Cooking Time: 10 minutes

Servings: 4

Ingredients:

- tablespoons plain yogurt
- ½ teaspoon red chili powder
- ¼ teaspoon ground cumin
- ¼ teaspoon ground turmeric
- Salt, to taste
- 1 lb. broccoli, cut into small florets
- tablespoons chickpea flour

Directions:

1 In an open bowl, mix together the yogurt, and spices.

2 Add the broccoli and coat with marinade generously.

3 Refrigerate for about 20 minutes.

4 Press the "Power Button" of Air Fry Oven and turn the dial to select the "Air Fry" mode.

5 Press the Time button and again turn the dial to set the cooking time to 10 minutes.

6 Now push the Temp button and rotate the dial to set the temperature at 400 degrees F.

7 Press the "Start/Pause" button to start.

8 When the unit beeps to show that it is preheated, open the lid.

9 Arrange the broccoli florets in "Air Fry Basket" and insert it in the oven.

10 Toss the broccoli florets once halfway through.

11 Serve warm.

Nutrition:

Calories 69 Total Fat 0.9 g

Saturated Fat 0.1 g

Cholesterol 0 mg

Sodium 87 mg

Total Carbs 12.2 g

Fiber 4.2 g

Sugar 3.2 g

Protein 4.9 g

159. Cheesy Broccoli Bites

Difficulty: Medium

Preparation Time: 15 minutes

Cooking Time: 12 minutes

Servings: 5

Ingredients:

- 1 cup broccoli florets
- 1 egg, beaten
- ¾ cup cheddar cheese, grated
- tablespoons Parmesan cheese, grated
- ¾ cup panko breadcrumbs
- Salt and freshly ground black pepper, as needed

Directions:

1 In a food processor, add the broccoli and pulse until finely crumbled.

2 In a large bowl, mix together the broccoli and remaining ingredients.

3 Make small equal-sized balls from the mixture.

4 Press the "Power Button" of Air Fry Oven and turn the dial to select the "Air Fry" mode.

5 Press the Time button and again turn the dial to set the cooking time to 12 minutes.

6 Now push the Temp button and rotate the dial to set the temperature at 350 degrees F.

7 Press the "Start/Pause" button to start.

8 When the unit beeps to show that it is preheated, open the lid.

9 Arrange the broccoli balls in "Air Fry Basket" and insert them in the oven.

10 Serve warm.

Nutrition:

Calories 153 Total Fat 8.2 g

Saturated Fat 4.5g Cholesterol 52 mg

Sodium 172 mg

Total Carbs 4 g

Fiber 0.5 g

Sugar 0.5 g

Protein 7.1 g

160. Mixed Veggie Bites

Difficulty: Medium

Preparation Time: 15 minutes

Cooking Time: 10 minutes

Servings: 5

Ingredients:

- ¾ lb. fresh spinach, blanched, drained, and chopped
- ¼ of onion, chopped
- ½ of carrot, peeled and chopped
- 1 garlic clove, minced
- 1 American cheese slice, cut into tiny pieces
- 1 bread slice, toasted and processed into breadcrumbs
- ½ tablespoon cornflour
- ½ teaspoon red chili flakes
- Salt, as required

Directions:

1 Place all ingredients in a bowl, except breadcrumbs, and mix until well combined.

2 Add the breadcrumbs and gently stir to combine.

3 Make 10 equal-sized balls from the mixture.

4 Press the "Power Button" of Air Fry Oven and turn the dial to select the "Air Fry" mode.

5 Press the Time button and again turn the dial to set the cooking time to 10 minutes.

6 Now push the Temp button and rotate the dial to set the temperature at 355 degrees F.

7 Press the "Start/Pause" button to start.

8 When the unit beeps to show that it is preheated, open the lid.

9 Arrange the veggie balls in "Air Fry Basket" and insert them in the oven.

10 Serve warm.

Nutrition:

Calories 43 Total Fat 1.4 g

Saturated Fat 0.7 g

Cholesterol 3 mg

Sodium 155 mg

Total Carbs 5.6 g

Fiber 1.9 g

Sugar 1.2 g

Protein 3.1 g

161. Risotto Bites

Difficulty: Medium

Preparation Time: 15 minutes

Cooking Time: 10 minutes

Servings: 4

Ingredients:

- 1½ cups cooked risotto
- tablespoons Parmesan cheese, grated
- ½ egg, beaten
- 1½ oz. mozzarella cheese, cubed
- 1/3 cup breadcrumbs

Directions:

1 In a bowl, add the risotto, Parmesan, and egg and mix until well combined.

2 Make 20 equal-sized balls from the mixture.

3 Insert a mozzarella cube in the center of each ball.

4 With your fingers, smooth the risotto mixture to cover the ball.

5 In a shallow dish, place the breadcrumbs.

6 Coat the balls with the breadcrumbs evenly.

7 Press the "Power Button" of Air Fry Oven and turn the dial to select the "Air Fry" mode.

8 Press the Time button and again turn the dial to set the cooking time to 10 minutes.

9 Now push the Temp button and rotate the dial to set the temperature at 390 degrees F.

10 Press the "Start/Pause" button to start.

11 When the unit beeps to show that it is preheated, open the lid.

12 Arrange the balls in "Air Fry Basket" and insert them in the oven.

13 Serve warm.

Nutrition:

Calories 340

Total Fat 4.3 g

Saturated Fat 2 g

Cholesterol 29 mg

Sodium 173 mg

Total Carbs 62.4 g

Fiber 1.3 g

Sugar 0.7 g

Protein 11.3 g

162. Rice Flour Bites

Difficulty: Medium

Preparation Time: 15 minutes

Cooking Time: 12 minutes

Servings: 4

Ingredients:

- tablespoons milk
- ½ teaspoon vegetable oil
- ¾ cup of rice flour
- 1 oz. Parmesan cheese, shredded

Directions:

1. In a bowl, add milk, flour, oil, and cheese and mix until a smooth dough forms.
2. Make small equal-sized balls from the dough.
3. Press the "Power Button" of Air Fry Oven and turn the dial to select the "Air Fry" mode.
4. Press the Time button and again turn the dial to set the cooking time to 12 minutes.
5. Now push the Temp button and rotate the dial to set the temperature at 300 degrees F.
6. Press the "Start/Pause" button to start.
7. When the unit beeps to show that it is preheated, open the lid.
8. Arrange the balls in "Air Fry Basket" and insert them in the oven.
9. Serve warm.

Nutrition:

Calories 148

Total Fat 3 g

Saturated Fat 1.5 g

Cholesterol 7 mg

Sodium 77 mg

Total Carbs 25.1 g

Fiber 0.7 g

Sugar 1.1 g

Protein 4.8 g

163. Lemon Parmesan and Peas Risotto

Difficulty: Hard

Preparation Time: 10 minutes

Cooking Time: 17 minutes

Servings: 6

Ingredients:

- tablespoons butter
- 1½ cup of rice
- 1 yellow onion, peeled and chopped
- 1 tablespoon extra-virgin olive oil
- 1 teaspoon lemon zest, grated
- 3½ cups chicken stock
- tablespoons lemon juice
- tablespoons parsley, diced
- tablespoons Parmesan cheese, finely grated
- Salt and ground black pepper, to taste
- 1½ cup peas

Directions:

1. Put the Instant Pot in the sauté mode, add 1 tablespoon of butter and oil, and heat them. Add the onion, mix, and cook for 5 minutes.
2. Add the rice, mix, and cook for another 3 minutes. Add 3 cups of broth and lemon juice, mix, cover, and cook for 5 minutes on rice.
3. Release the pressure, put the fryer in manual mode, add the peas and the rest of the broth, stir and cook for 2 minutes.

4 Add the cheese, parsley, remaining butter, lemon zest, salt, and pepper to taste and mix. Divide between plates and serve.

Nutrition:

Calories: 140,

Fat: 1.5

Fiber: 1,

Carbohydrate: 27,

Proteins: 5

164. Spinach and Goat Cheese Risotto

Difficulty: Hard

Preparation Time: 10 minutes

Cooking Time: 10 minutes

Servings: 6

Ingredients:

- ¾ cup yellow onion, chopped
- 1½ cups Arborio rice
- ounces spinach, chopped
- 3½ cups hot vegetable stock
- ½ cup white wine
- garlic cloves, peeled and minced
- tablespoons extra virgin olive oil
- Salt and ground black pepper, to taste
- 1/3 cup pecans, toasted and chopped
- ounces goat cheese, soft and crumbled
- tablespoons lemon juice

Directions:

1 Put the Instant Pot in the sauté mode, add the oil and heat. Add garlic and onion, mix and cook for 5 minutes.

2 Add the rice, mix, and cook for 1 minute. Add wine, stir and cook until it is absorbed. Add 3 cups of stock, cover the Instant Pot, and cook the rice for 4 minutes.

3 Release the pressure, uncover the Instant Pot, add the spinach, stir and cook for 3 minutes in Manual mode. Add salt, pepper, the rest of the stock, lemon juice, and goat cheese and mix. Divide between plates, decorate with nuts, and serve.

Nutrition:

Calories: 340,

Fat: 23,

Fiber: 4.5,

Carbohydrate: 24,

Proteins: 18.9

165. Rice and Artichokes

Difficulty: Hard

Preparation Time: 10 minutes

Cooking Time: 20 minutes

Servings: 4

Ingredients:

- garlic cloves, peeled and crushed
- 1¼ cups chicken broth
- 1 tablespoon extra-virgin olive oil
- ounces Arborio rice

- 1 tablespoon white wine
- ounces canned artichoke hearts, chopped
- ounces cream cheese
- 1 tablespoon grated Parmesan cheese
- 1½ tablespoons fresh thyme, chopped
- Salt and ground black pepper, to taste
- ounces graham cracker crumbs
- 1¼ cups water

Directions:

1 Put the Instant Pot in the sauté mode, add the oil, heat, add the rice, and cook for 2 minutes. Add the garlic, mix, and cook for 1 minute.

2 Transfer to a heat-resistant plate. Add the stock, crumbs, salt, pepper, wine, mix, and cover the dish with aluminum foil.

3 Place the dish in the basket to cook the Instant Pot, add water, cover, and cook for 8 minutes on rice. Release the pressure, remove the plate, uncover, and add cream cheese, parmesan, artichoke hearts, and thyme.

4 Mix well and serve.

Nutrition:

Calories: 240,

Fat: 7.2

Fiber: 5.1

Carbohydrate: 34,

Proteins: 6

166. Potatoes Au Gratin

Difficulty: Hard

Preparation Time: 10 minutes

Cooking Time: 17 minutes

Servings: 6

Ingredients:

- ½ cup yellow onion, chopped
- tablespoons butter
- 1 cup chicken stock
- potatoes, peeled and sliced
- ½ cup sour cream
- Salt and ground black pepper, to taste
- 1 cup Monterey jack cheese, shredded
- For the topping:
- tablespoons melted butter
- 1 cup breadcrumbs

Directions:

1 Put the Instant Pot in Saute mode, add the butter and melt. Add the onion, mix and cook for 5 minutes. Add the stock, salt and pepper and put the steamer basket in the Instant Pot also.

2 Add the potatoes, cover the Instant Pot and cook for 5 minutes in the Manual setting. In a bowl, mix 3 tablespoons of butter with breadcrumbs and mix well. Relieve the pressure of the Instant Pot, remove the steam basket and transfer the potatoes to a pan.

3 Pour the cream and cheese into the instant pot and mix. Add the potatoes and mix gently.

4 Spread breadcrumbs, mix everywhere, place on a preheated grill and cook for 7 minutes. Let cool for more minutes and serve.

Nutrition:

Calories: 340,

Fat: 22,

Fiber: 2,

Carbohydrate: 32,

Proteins: 11

CHAPTER 9:

Snacks

167. Sweet Potato Tater Tots

Difficulty: Very Easy

Preparation Time: 10 minutes.

Cooking Time: 23 minutes

Servings: 4

Ingredients:

- sweet potatoes, peeled
- 1/2 tsp. Cajun seasoning
- Olive oil cooking spray
- Sea salt to taste

Directions:

1 Boil sweet potatoes in water for 15 minutes over medium-high heat.

2 Drain the sweet potatoes then allow them to cool

3 Peel the boiled sweet potatoes and return them to the bowl.

4 Mash the potatoes and stir in salt and Cajun seasoning. Mix well and make small tater tots out of it.

5 Place the tater tots in the Air Fryer basket and spray them with cooking oil.

6 Place the Air Fryer basket inside the Air Fryer toaster and close the lid.

7 Select Air Frying mode at a temperature of 400 ° F for 8 minutes.

8 Turn the trays over and continue cooking for another 8 minutes.

9 Serve fresh.

Nutrition:

Calories: 184 Cal

Protein: 9 g

Carbs: 43 g

Fat: 17 g

168. Fried Ravioli

Difficulty: Hard

Preparation Time: 10 minutes

Cooking Time: 15 minutes

Servings: 4

Ingredients:

- 1 package ravioli, frozen
- 1 cup breadcrumbs
- 1/2 cup parmesan cheese
- 1 tbs. Italian seasoning
- 1 tbs. garlic powder
- eggs, beaten
- Cooking spray

Directions:

1 Mix breadcrumbs with garlic powder, cheese, and Italian seasoning in a bowl.

2 Whisk eggs in another bowl. Dip each ravioli in eggs first then coat them with crumbs mixture.

3 Place the ravioli in the Air Fryer basket. Place the air Fryer basket inside the oven and close the lid.
4 Select the Air Fry mode at 360°F temperature for 15 minutes.
5 Flip the ravioli after 8 minutes and resume cooking. Serve warm.

Nutrition:

Calories: 124 Cal

Protein: 4.5 g

Carbs: 27.5 g

Fat: 3.5 g

169. Eggplant Fries

Difficulty: Very Easy

Preparation Time: 10 minutes

Cooking Time: 20 minutes

Servings: 4

Ingredients:

- 1/2 cup panko breadcrumbs
- 1/2 tsp. salt
- 1 eggplant, peeled and sliced
- 1 cup egg, whisked

Directions:

1 Toss the breadcrumbs with salt in a tray.
2 Dip the eggplant in the whisked egg and coat with the crumb's mixture.
3 Place the eggplant slices in the Air Fryer basket. Put the basket inside the Air Fryer toaster oven and close the lid.
4 Select the Air Fry mode at 400°F temperature for 20 minutes.
5 Flip the slices after 10 minutes then resume cooking. Serve warm.

Nutrition:

Calories: 110 Cal Protein: 5 g

Carbs: 12.8 g Fat: 11.9 g

170. Stuffed Eggplants

Difficulty: Very Easy

Preparation Time: 10 minutes

Cooking Time: 38 minutes

Servings: 4

Ingredients:

- eggplants, cut in half lengthwise
- 1/2 cup shredded cheddar cheese
- 1/2 can (7.5 oz.) chili without beans
- tsp. kosher salt
- FOR SERVING
- tbsp. cooked bacon bits
- tbsp. sour cream
- Fresh scallions, thinly sliced

Directions:

1 Place the eggplants halves in the Air Fryer toaster oven and close the lid.
2 Select the Air Fry mode at 390°F temperature for 35 minutes.
3 Top each eggplant half with chili, cheese, and salt.
4 Place the halves in a baking pan and return to the oven. Select the Broil mode at 375°F temperature for 3 minutes.
5 Garnish with bacon bits, sour cream, and scallions. Serve.

Nutrition:

Calories: 113 Cal Protein: 9.2 g

Carbs: 13 g Fat: 21 g

171. Bacon Poppers

Difficulty: Very Easy

Preparation Time: 10 minutes

Cooking Time: 15 minutes

Servings: 4

Ingredients:

- strips bacon, crispy cooked
- Dough:
- 2/3 cup water
- tbsp. butter
- 1 tbsp. bacon fat
- 1 tsp. kosher salt
- 2/3 cup all-purpose flour
- eggs
- oz. Cheddar cheese, shredded
- ½ cup jalapeno peppers
- A pinch pepper
- A pinch black pepper

Directions:

1 Whisk butter with water and salt in a skillet over medium heat. Stir in flour, then stir cook for about 3 minutes.

2 Transfer this flour to a bowl, then whisk in eggs and rest of the ingredients.

3 Fold in bacon and mix well. Wrap this dough in a plastic sheet and refrigerate for 30 minutes. Make small balls out of this dough.

4 Place these bacon balls the Air Fryer toaster oven and close the lid.

5 Select the Air Fry mode at 390°F temperature for 15 minutes. Flip the balls after 7 minutes then resume cooking. Serve warm.

Nutrition:

Calories: 240 Cal

Protein: 14.9 g

Carbs: 7.1 g

Fat: 22.5 g

172. Stuffed Jalapeno

Difficulty: Very Easy

Preparation Time: 10 minutes

Cooking Time: 10 minutes

Servings: 4

Ingredients:

- 1 lb. ground pork sausage
- 1 (8 oz.) package cream cheese, softened
- 1 cup shredded Parmesan cheese
- 1 lb. large fresh jalapeno peppers halved lengthwise and seeded
- 1 (8 oz.) bottle Ranch dressing

Directions:

1 Mix pork sausage ground with ranch dressing and cream cheese in a bowl.

2 But the jalapeno in half and remove their seeds.

3 Divide the cream cheese mixture into the jalapeno halves. Place the jalapeno pepper in a baking tray.

4 Set the Baking tray inside the Air Fryer toaster oven and close the lid.

5 Select the Bake mode at 350°F temperature for 10 minutes. Serve warm.

Nutrition:

Calories: 168 Cal Protein: 9.4 g

Carbs: 12.1 g Fat: 21.2 g

173. Creamy Mushrooms

Difficulty: Very Easy

Preparation Time: 10 minutes

Cooking Time: 15 minutes

Servings: 24

Ingredients:

- 20 mushrooms
- 1 orange bell pepper, dice d
- 1 onion, diced
- slices bacon, diced
- 1 cup shredded Cheddar cheese
- 1 cup sour cream

Directions:

1 First sauté the mushroom stems, with onion, bacon, and bell pepper in a pan.

2 After 5 minutes of cooking, add 1 cup cheese and sour cream. Cook for 2 minutes.

3 Place the mushroom caps on the Air Fryer basket crisper plate.

4 Stuff each mushroom with the cheese-vegetable mixture and top them with cheddar cheese.

5 Insert the basket back insider and select Air Fry mode for 8 minutes at 350°F.

6 Serve warm.

Nutrition:

Calories: 101 Cal

Protein: 8.8 g

Carbs: 25 g

Fat: 12.2 g

174. Italian Corn Fritters

Difficulty: Very Easy

Preparation Time: 10 minutes

Cooking Time: 3 minutes

Servings: 4

Ingredients:

- cups frozen corn kernels
- 1/3 cup finely ground cornmeal
- 1/3 cup flour
- ½ tsp. salt
- ¼ tsp. pepper
- ½ tsp. baking powder
- Onion powder, to taste
- Garlic powder, to taste
- ¼ tsp. paprika
- tbsp. green chilies with juices
- tbsp. almond milk
- ¼ cup chopped Italian parsley

Directions:

1 Beat cornmeal with flour, baking powder, parsley, seasonings in a bowl. Blend 3 tbsp. almond milk with 1 cup corn, black pepper, and salt in a food processor until smooth.

2 Stir in the flour mixture then mix until smooth. Spread this corn mixture in a baking tray, lined with wax paper.

3 Set the baking tray inside the Air Fryer toaster oven and close the lid.

4 Select the bake mode at 350°F temperature for 2 minutes. Slice and serve.

Nutrition:

Calories: 146 Cal Protein: 6.3 g

Carbs: 18.8 g Fat: 4.5 g

175. Artichoke Fries

Difficulty: Very Easy

Preparation Time: 8 minutes

Cooking Time: 13 minutes

Servings: 6

Ingredients:

- 1 oz. can artichoke hearts
- 1 cup flour
- 1 cup almond milk
- ½ tsp. garlic powder
- ¾ tsp. salt
- ¼ tsp. black pepper, or to taste
- For Dry Mix:
- 1 ½ cup panko breadcrumbs
- ½ tsp. paprika
- ¼ tsp. salt

Directions:

1 Whisk the wet ingredients in a bowl until smooth and mix the dry ingredients in a separate bowl.

2 First, dip the artichokes quarters in the wet mixture then coat with the dry panko mixture.

3 Place the artichokes hearts in the Air Fryer basket. Insert the basket inside the Air Fryer toaster oven and close the lid.

4 Select the Air Fry mode at 340°F temperature for 13 minutes. Serve warm.

Nutrition:

Calories: 199 Cal

Protein: 9.4 g

Carbs: 15.9 g

Fat: 4 g

176. Crumbly Beef Meatballs

Difficulty: Very Easy

Preparation Time: 8 minutes

Cooking Time: 20 minutes

Servings: 6

Ingredients:

- lbs. of ground beef
- large eggs
- 1-1/4 cup panko breadcrumbs
- 1/4 cup chopped fresh parsley
- 1 tsp. dried oregano
- 1/4 cup grated Parmigianino Reggiano
- 1 small clove garlic chopped
- salt and pepper to taste
- 1 tsp. vegetable oil

Directions:

1 Thoroughly mix beef with eggs, crumbs, parsley, and rest of the ingredients.

2 Make small meatballs out of this mixture and place them in the basket.

3 Place the basket inside the Air Fryer toaster oven and close the lid.

4 Select the Air Fry mode at 350°F temperature for 13 minutes.

5 Toss the meatballs after 5 minutes and resume cooking.

6 Serve fresh.

Nutrition:

Calories: 221 Cal

Protein: 25.1 g

Carbs: 11.2 g

Fat: 16.5 g

177. Pork Stuffed Dumplings

Difficulty: Very Easy

Preparation Time: 15 minutes

Cooking Time: 12 minutes

Servings: 3

Ingredients:

- 1 tsp. canola oil
- cups chopped book Choy
- 1 tbsp. chopped fresh ginger
- 1 tbsp. chopped garlic
- oz. ground pork
- 1/4 tsp. crushed red pepper
- 18 dumpling wrappers
- Cooking spray
- tbsp. rice vinegar
- tsp. lower-sodium soy sauce
- 1 tsp. toasted sesame oil
- 1/2 tsp. packed light Sugar
- 1 tbsp. finely chopped scallions

Directions:

1 In a greased skillet, sauté bok choy for 8 minutes, then add ginger and garlic. Cook for 1 minute.
2 Transfer the bok choy to a plate.
3 Add pork and red pepper then mix well. Place the dumpling wraps on the working surface and divide the pork fillings on the dumpling wraps.
4 Wet the edges of the wraps and pinch them together to seal the filling.
5 Place the dumpling in the Air Fryer basket.
6 Set the Air Fryer basket inside the Air Fryer toaster oven and close the lid.
7 Select the Air Fry mode at 375°F temperature for 12 minutes.
8 Flip the dumplings after 6 minutes then resume cooking.
9 Serve fresh.

Nutrition:

Calories: 172 Cal

Protein: 2.1 g

Carbs: 18.6 g

Fat: 10.7 g

178. Panko Tofu with Mayo Sauce

Difficulty: Very Easy

Preparation Time: 10 minutes

Cooking Time: 20 minutes

Servings: 4

Ingredients:

- tofu cutlets
- For the Marinade
- 1 tbsp toasted sesame oil
- 1/4 cup soy sauce
- 1 tsp rice vinegar
- 1/2 tsp garlic powder
- 1 tsp. ground ginger
- Make the Tofu:
- 1/2 cup vegan mayo
- 1 cup panko breadcrumbs
- 1 tsp. of sea salt

Directions:

1 Whisk the marinade ingredients in a bowl and add tofu cutlets. Mix well to coat the cutlets.
2 Cover and marinate for 1 hour. Meanwhile, whisk crumbs with salt and mayo in a bowl.

3 Coat the cutlets with crumbs mixture. Place the tofu cutlets in the Air Fryer basket.
4 Select the Air Fry mode at 370°F temperature for 20 minutes. Flip the cutlets after 10 minutes then resume cooking.
5 Serve warm.

Nutrition:

Calories: 151 Cal Protein: 1.9 g

Carbs: 6.9 g Fat: 8.6 g

179. Garlicky Bok Choy

Difficulty: Very Easy

Preparation Time: 10 minutes

Cooking Time: 10 minutes

Servings: 2

Ingredients:

- bunches baby book Choy
- Spray oil
- 1 tsp. garlic powder

Directions:

1 Toss bok choy with garlic powder and spread them in the Air Fryer basket.
2 Spray them with cooking oil.
3 Place the basket inside the Air Fryer toaster oven and close the lid.
4 Select the Air Fry mode at 350°F temperature for 6 minutes. Serve fresh.

Nutrition:

Calories: 81 Cal Protein: 0.4 g

Carbs: 4.7 g Fat: 8.3 g

180. Soda Bread

Difficulty: Very Easy

Preparation Time: 15 minutes

Cooking Time: 30 minutes

Servings: 10

Ingredients:

- cups whole-wheat flour
- 1 tablespoon sugar
- teaspoon caraway seeds
- 1 teaspoon baking soda
- 1 teaspoon sea salt
- ¼ cup chilled butter, cubed into small pieces
- 1 large egg, beaten
- 1½ cups buttermilk

Directions:

1 In a large bowl, mix the flour, sugar, caraway seeds, baking soda, salt, and mix well.

2 With a pastry cutter, cut in the butter flour until coarse crumbs like mixture is formed.

3 Make a well in the center of flour mixture.

4 In the well, add the egg, followed by the buttermilk and with a spatula, mix until well combined.

5 With floured hand, shape the dough into a ball.

6 Place the dough onto a floured surface and lightly need it.

7 Shape the dough into a 6-inch ball.

8 With a serrated knife, score an X on the top of the dough.

9 Press "Power Button" of Air Fry Oven and turn the dial to select the "Air Crisp" mode.

10 Press the Time button and again turn the dial to set the cooking time to 30 minutes

11 Now push the Temp button and rotate the dial to set the temperature at 350 degrees F.

12 Press "Start/Pause" button to start.

13 When the unit beeps to show that it is preheated, open the lid.

14 Arrange the dough in lightly greased "Air Fry Basket" and insert in the oven. Place the pan onto a wire rack to cool for about 10 minutes

15 Carefully, invert the bread onto wire rack to cool completely before slicing.

16 Cut the bread into desired-sized slices and serve.

Nutrition:

Calories 205 Fat 5.9 g Carbs 31.8 g Protein 5.9 g

181. Baguette Bread

Difficulty: Very Easy

Preparation Time: 15 minutes

Cooking Time: 20 minutes

Servings: 8

Ingredients:

- ¾ cup warm water
- ¾ teaspoon quick yeast
- ½ teaspoon demerara sugar
- 1 cup bread flour
- ½ cup whole-wheat flour
- ½ cup oat flour
- 1¼ teaspoons salt

Directions:

1 In a large bowl, place the water and sprinkle with yeast and sugar.

2 Set aside for 5 minutes or until foamy.

3 Add the bread flour and salt mix until a stiff dough form.

4 Put the dough onto a floured surface and with your hands, knead until smooth and elastic.

5 Now, shape the dough into a ball.

6 Place the dough into a slightly oiled bowl and turn to coat well.

7 With a plastic wrap, cover the bowl and place in a warm place for about 1 hour or until doubled in size.

8 With your hands, punch down the dough and form into a long slender loaf.

9 Place the loaf onto a lightly greased baking sheet and set aside in warm place, uncovered, for about 30 minutes

10 Press "Power Button" of Air Fry Oven and turn the dial to select the "Air Bake" mode.

11 Press the Time button and again turn the dial to set the cooking time to 20 minutes

12 Now push the Temp button and rotate the dial to set the temperature at 450 degrees F.

13 Press "Start/Pause" button to start.

14 When the unit beeps to show that it is preheated, open the lid.

15 Carefully, arrange the dough onto the "Wire Rack" and insert in the oven.

16 Carefully, invert the bread onto wire rack to cool completely before slicing.

17 Cut the bread into desired-sized slices and serve.

Nutrition:

Calories 114

Fat 0.8 g

Carbs 22.8 g

Protein 3.8 g

182. Yogurt Bread

Difficulty: Very Easy

Preparation Time: 20 minutes

Cooking Time: 40 minutes

Servings: 10

Ingredients:

- 1½ cups warm water, divided
- 1½ teaspoons active dry yeast
- 1 teaspoon sugar
- cups all-purpose flour
- 1 cup plain Greek yogurt
- teaspoons kosher salt

Directions:

1 Add ½ cup of the warm water, yeast and sugar in the bowl of a stand mixer, fitted with the dough hook attachment and mix well.

2 Set aside for about 5 minutes

3 Add the flour, yogurt, and salt and mix on medium-low speed until the dough comes together.

4 Then, mix on medium speed for 5 minutes

5 Place the dough into a bowl.

6 With a plastic wrap, cover the bowl and place in a warm place for about 2-3 hours or until doubled in size.

7 Transfer the dough onto a lightly floured surface and shape into a smooth ball.

8 Place the dough onto a greased parchment paper-lined rack.

9 With a kitchen towel, cover the dough and let rest for 15 minutes

10 With a very sharp knife, cut a 4x½-inch deep cut down the center of the dough.

11 Press "Power Button" of Air Fry Oven and turn the dial to select the "Air Roast" mode.

12 Press the Time button and again turn the dial to set the cooking time to 40 minutes

13 Now push the Temp button and rotate the dial to set the temperature at 325 degrees F.

14 Press "Start/Pause" button to start.

15 When the unit beeps to show that it is preheated, open the lid.

16 Carefully, arrange the dough onto the "Wire Rack" and insert in the oven.

17 Carefully, invert the bread onto wire rack to cool completely before slicing.

18 Cut the bread into desired-sized slices and serve.

Nutrition:

Calories 157 Fat 0.7 g Carbs 31 g Protein 5.5 g

183. Sunflower Seed Bread

Difficulty: Very Easy

Preparation Time: 15 minutes

Cooking Time: 18 minutes

Servings: 6

Ingredients:

- 2/3 cup whole-wheat flour
- 2/3 cup plain flour
- 1/3 cup sunflower seeds
- ½ sachet instant yeast
- 1 teaspoon salt
- 2/3-1 cup lukewarm water

Directions:

1 In a bowl, mix the flours, sunflower seeds, yeast, and salt.

2 Slowly, add in the water, stirring continuously until a soft dough ball form.

3 Now, move the dough onto a lightly floured surface and knead for about 5 minutes using your hands.

4 Make a ball from the dough and place into a bowl.

5 With a plastic wrap, cover the bowl and place at a warm place for about 30 minutes

6 Grease a cake pan.

7 Coat the top of dough with water and place into the prepared cake pan.

8 Press "Power Button" of Air Fry Oven and turn the dial to select the "Air Crisp" mode.

9 Press the Time button and again turn the dial to set the cooking time to 18 minutes

10 Now push the Temp button and rotate the dial to set the temperature at 390 degrees F.

11 Press "Start/Pause" button to start.

12 When the unit beeps to show that it is preheated, open the lid.

13 Arrange the pan in "Air Fry Basket" and insert in the oven.

14 Place the pan onto a wire rack to cool for about 10 minutes

15 Carefully, invert the bread onto wire rack to cool completely before slicing.

16 Cut the bread into desired-sized slices and serve.

Nutrition:

Calories 132

Fat 1.7 g

Carbs 24.4 g

Protein 4.9 g

184. Date Bread

Difficulty: Very Easy

Preparation Time: 15 minutes

Cooking Time: 22 minutes

Servings: 10

Ingredients:

- 2½ cup dates, pitted and chopped
- ¼ cup butter
- 1 cup hot water
- 1½ cups flour
- ½ cup brown sugar
- 1 teaspoon baking powder
- 1 teaspoon baking soda
- ½ teaspoon salt
- 1 egg

Directions:

1 In a large bowl, add the dates, butter and top with the hot water.

2 Set aside for about 5 minutes

3 In another bowl, mix the flour, brown sugar, baking powder, baking soda, and salt.

4 In the same bowl of dates, mix well the flour mixture, and egg.

5 Grease a baking pan.

6 Place the mixture into the prepared pan.

7 Press "Power Button" of Air Fry Oven and turn the dial to select the "Air Crisp" mode.

8 Press the Time button and again turn the dial to set the cooking time to 22 minutes

9 Now push the Temp button and rotate the dial to set the temperature at 340 degrees F.

10 Press "Start/Pause" button to start.

11 When the unit beeps to show that it is preheated, open the lid.

12 Arrange the pan in "Air Fry Basket" and insert in the oven.

13 Place the pan onto a wire rack to cool for about 10 minutes

14 Carefully, invert the bread onto wire rack to cool completely before slicing.

15 Cut the bread into desired-sized slices and serve.

Nutrition:

Calories 269

Fat 5.4 g

Carbs 55.1 g

Protein 3.6 g

185. Date & Walnut Bread

Difficulty: Very Easy

Preparation Time: 15 minutes

Cooking Time: 35 minutes

Servings: 5

Ingredients:

- 1 cup dates, pitted and sliced
- ¾ cup walnuts, chopped
- 1 tablespoon instant coffee powder

- 1 tablespoon hot water
- 1¼ cups plain flour
- ¼ teaspoon salt
- ½ teaspoon baking powder
- ½ teaspoon baking soda
- ½ cup condensed milk
- ½ cup butter, softened
- ½ teaspoon vanilla essence

Directions:

1. In a large bowl, add the dates, butter and top with the hot water.
2. Set aside for about 30 minutes
3. Dry out well and set aside.
4. In a small bowl, add the coffee powder and hot water and mix well.
5. In a large bowl, mix the flour, baking powder, baking soda and salt.
6. In another large bowl, add the condensed milk and butter and beat until smooth.
7. Add the flour mixture, coffee mixture and vanilla essence and mix until well combined.
8. Fold in dates and ½ cup of walnut.
9. Line a baking pan with a lightly greased parchment paper.
10. Place the mixture into the prepared pan and sprinkle with the remaining walnuts.
11. Press "Power Button" of Air Fry Oven and turn the dial to select the "Air Crisp" mode.
12. Press the Time button and again turn the dial to set the cooking time to 35 minutes
13. Now push the Temp button and rotate the dial to set the temperature at 320 degrees F.
14. Press "Start/Pause" button to start.
15. When the unit beeps to show that it is preheated, open the lid.
16. Arrange the pan in "Air Fry Basket" and insert in the oven.
17. Place the pan onto a wire rack to cool for about 10 minutes
18. Carefully, invert the bread onto wire rack to cool completely before slicing.
19. Cut the bread into desired-sized slices and serve.

Nutrition:

Calories 593 Fat 32.6 g

Carbs 69.4 g Protein 11.2 g

186. Brown Sugar Banana Bread

Difficulty: Easy

Preparation Time: 15 minutes

Cooking Time: 30 minutes

Servings: 4

Ingredients:

- 1 egg
- 1 ripe banana, peeled and mashed
- ¼ cup milk
- tablespoons canola oil

- tablespoons brown sugar
- ¾ cup plain flour
- ½ teaspoon baking soda

Directions:

- Line a very small baking pan with a greased parchment paper.
- In a small bowl, add the egg and banana and beat well.
- Add the milk, oil and sugar and beat until well combined.
- Add the flour and baking soda and mix until just combined.
- Place the mixture into prepared pan.
- Press "Power Button" of Air Fry Oven and turn the dial to select the "Air Crisp" mode.
- Press the Time button and again turn the dial to set the cooking time to 30 minutes
- Now push the Temp button and rotate the dial to set the temperature at 320 degrees F.
- Press "Start/Pause" button to start.
- When the unit beeps to show that it is preheated, open the lid.
- Arrange the pan in "Air Fry Basket" and insert in the oven.
- Place the pan onto a wire rack to cool for about 10 minutes
- Carefully, invert the bread onto wire rack to cool completely before slicing.
- Cut the bread into desired-sized slices and serve.

Nutrition:

Calories 214

Fat 8.7 g

Carbs 29.9 g

Protein 4.6 g

187. Cinnamon Banana Bread

Difficulty: Easy

Preparation Time: 15 minutes

Cooking Time: 20 minutes

Servings: 8

Ingredients:

- 1 1/3 cups flour
- 2/3 cup sugar
- 1 teaspoon baking soda
- 1 teaspoon baking powder
- 1 teaspoon ground cinnamon
- 1 teaspoon salt
- ½ cup milk
- ½ cup olive oil
- bananas, peeled and sliced

Directions:

1. In the bowl of a stand mixer, add all the ingredients and mix well.
2. Grease a loaf pan.
3. Place the mixture into the prepared pan.
4. Press "Power Button" of Air Fry Oven and turn the dial to select the "Air Crisp" mode.

5 Press the Time button and again turn the dial to set the cooking time to 20 minutes

6 Now push the Temp button and rotate the dial to set the temperature at 330 degrees F.

7 Press "Start/Pause" button to start.

8 When the unit beeps to show that it is preheated, open the lid.

9 Arrange the pan in "Air Fry Basket" and insert in the oven.

10 Place the pan onto a wire rack to cool for about 10 minutes

11 Carefully, invert the bread onto wire rack to cool completely before slicing.

12 Cut the bread into desired-sized slices and serve.

Nutrition:

Calories 295 Fat 13.3g Carbs 44 g Protein 3.1 g

188. Banana & Walnut Bread

Difficulty: Easy

Preparation Time: 15 minutes

Cooking Time: 25 minutes

Servings: 10

Ingredients:

1½ cups self-rising flour

¼ teaspoon bicarbonate of soda

5 tablespoons plus 1 teaspoon butter

2/3 cup plus ½ tablespoon caster sugar

2 medium eggs

3½ oz. walnuts, chopped

2 cups bananas, peeled and mashed

Directions:

In a bowl, mix the flour and bicarbonate of soda.

In another bowl, add the butter, and sugar and beat until pale and fluffy.

Add the eggs, one at a time along with a little flour and mix well.

Stir in the remaining flour and walnuts.

Add the bananas and mix until well combined.

Grease a loaf pan.

Place the mixture into the prepared pan.

Press "Power Button" of Air Fry Oven and turn the dial to select the "Air Crisp" mode.

Press the Time button and again turn the dial to set the cooking time to 10 minutes

Now push the Temp button and rotate the dial to set the temperature at 355 degrees F.

Press "Start/Pause" button to start.

When the unit beeps to show that it is preheated, open the lid.

Arrange the pan in "Air Fry Basket" and insert in the oven.

After 10 minutes of cooking, set the temperature at 338 degrees F for 15 minutes

Place the pan onto a wire rack to cool for about 10 minutes

Carefully, invert the bread onto wire rack to cool completely before slicing.

Cut the bread into desired-sized slices and serve.

Nutrition:

Calories 270 Fat 12.8 g Carbs 35.5 g Protein 5.8 g

189. Banana & Raisin Bread

Difficulty: Easy

Preparation Time: 15 minutes

Cooking Time: 40 minutes

Servings: 6

Ingredients:

- 1½ cups cake flour
- 1 teaspoon baking soda
- ½ teaspoon ground cinnamon
- Salt, to taste
- ½ cup vegetable oil
- eggs
- ½ cup sugar
- ½ teaspoon vanilla extract
- medium bananas, peeled and mashed
- ½ cup raisins, chopped finely

Directions:

1 In a large bowl, mix the flour, baking soda, cinnamon, and salt.

2 In another bowl, beat well eggs and oil.

3 Add the sugar, vanilla extract, and bananas and beat until well combined.

4 Add the flour mixture and stir until just combined.

5 Place the mixture into a lightly greased baking pan and sprinkle with raisins.

6 With a piece of foil, cover the pan loosely.

7 Press "Power Button" of Air Fry Oven and turn the dial to select the "Air Bake" mode.

8 Press the Time button and again turn the dial to set the cooking time to 30 minutes

9 Now push the Temp button and rotate the dial to set the temperature at 300 degrees F.

10 Press "Start/Pause" button to start.

11 When the unit beeps to show that it is preheated, open the lid.

12 Arrange the pan in "Air Fry Basket" and insert in the oven.

13 After 30 minutes of cooking, set the temperature to 285 degrees F for 10 minutes

14 Place the pan onto a wire rack to cool for about 10 minutes

15 Carefully, invert the bread onto wire rack to cool completely before slicing.

16 Cut the bread into desired-sized slices and serve.

Nutrition:

Calories 448 Fat 20.2 g Carbs 63.9 g Protein 6.1 g

190. 3-Ingredients Banana Bread

Difficulty: Medium

Preparation Time: 10 minutes

Cooking Time: 20 minutes

Servings: 6

Ingredients:

2 (6.4-oz.) banana muffin mix

1 cup water

1 ripe banana, peeled and mashed

Directions:

In a bowl, add all the ingredients and with a whisk, mix until well combined.

Place the mixture into a lightly greased loaf pan.

Press "Power Button" of Air Fry Oven and turn the dial to select the "Air Bake" mode.

Press the Time button and again turn the dial to set the cooking time to 20 minutes

Now push the Temp button and rotate the dial to set the temperature at 360 degrees F.

Press "Start/Pause" button to start.

When the unit beeps to show that it is preheated, open the lid.

Arrange the pan in "Air Fry Basket" and insert in the oven.

Place the pan onto a wire rack to cool for about 10 minutes

Carefully, invert the bread onto wire rack to cool completely before slicing. Cut the bread into desired-sized slices and serve.

Nutrition:

Calories 144 Fat 3.8 g Carbs 25.5 g Protein 1.9 g

191. Yogurt Banana Bread

Difficulty: Medium

Preparation Time: 15 minutes

Cooking Time: 28 minutes

Servings: 5

Ingredients:

- 1 medium very ripe banana, peeled and mashed
- 1 large egg
- 1 tablespoon canola oil
- 1 tablespoon plain Greek yogurt
- ¼ teaspoon pure vanilla extract
- ½ cup all-purpose flour
- ¼ cup granulated white sugar
- ¼ teaspoon ground cinnamon
- ¼ teaspoon baking soda
- 1/8 teaspoon sea salt

Directions:

1 In a bowl, add the mashed banana, egg, oil, yogurt, vanilla, and beat until well combined.

2 Add the flour, sugar, baking soda, cinnamon and salt and mix until just combined.

3 Place the mixture into a lightly greased mini loaf pan.

4 Press "Power Button" of Air Fry Oven and turn the dial to select the "Air Bake" mode.

5 Press the Time button and again turn the dial to set the cooking time to 28 minutes

6 Now push the Temp button and rotate the dial to set the temperature at 350 degrees F.

7 Press "Start/Pause" button to start.

8 When the unit beeps to show that it is preheated, open the lid.

9 Arrange the pan in "Air Fry Basket" and insert in the oven.

10 Place the pan onto a wire rack to cool for about 10 minutes

11 Carefully, invert the bread onto wire rack to cool completely before slicing.

12 Cut the bread into desired-sized slices and serve.

Nutrition:

Calories 145

Fat 4 g

Carbs 25 g

Protein 3 g

192. Sour Cream Banana Bread

Difficulty: Medium

Preparation Time: 15 minutes

Cooking Time: 37 minutes

Servings: 8

Ingredients:

- ¾ cup all-purpose flour
- ¼ teaspoon baking soda
- ¼ teaspoon salt
- ripe bananas, peeled and mashed
- ½ cup granulated sugar
- ¼ cup sour cream
- ¼ cup vegetable oil
- 1 large egg
- ½ teaspoon pure vanilla extract

Directions:

- In a large bowl, mix the flour, baking soda and salt.
- In another bowl, add the bananas, egg, sugar, sour cream, oil and vanilla and beat until well combined.
- Add the flour mixture and mix until just combined.
- Place the mixture into a lightly greased pan. Press "Power Button" of Air Fry Oven and turn the dial to select the "Air Crisp" mode.
- Press the Time button and again turn the dial to set the cooking time to 37 minutes
- Now push the Temp button and rotate the dial to set the temperature at 310 degrees F. Press "Start/Pause" button to start.
- When the unit beeps to show that it is preheated, open the lid. Arrange the pan in "Air Fry Basket" and insert in the oven.
- Place the pan onto a wire rack to cool for about 10 minutes
- Carefully, invert the bread onto wire rack to cool completely before slicing.
- Cut the bread into desired-sized slices and serve.

Nutrition:

Calories 201

Fat 9.2g

Carbs 28.6g

Protein 2.6g

193. Peanut Butter Banana Bread

Difficulty: Medium

Preparation Time: 15 minutes

Cooking Time: 40 minutes

Servings: 6

Ingredients:

- 1 cup plus 1 tablespoon all-purpose flour
- ¼ teaspoon baking soda
- 1 teaspoon baking powder
- ¼ teaspoon salt
- 1 large egg
- 1/3 cup granulated sugar
- ¼ cup canola oil
- tablespoons creamy peanut butter
- tablespoons sour cream
- 1 teaspoon vanilla extract
- medium ripe bananas, peeled and mashed
- ¾ cup walnuts, roughly chopped

Directions:

1. In a bowl and mix the flour, baking powder, baking soda, and salt.
2. In another large bowl, add the egg, sugar, oil, peanut butter, sour cream, and vanilla extract and beat until well combined.
3. Add the bananas and beat until well combined.
4. Add the flour mixture and mix until just combined.
5. Gently, fold in the walnuts.
6. Place the mixture into a lightly greased pan.
7. Press "Power Button" of Air Fry Oven and turn the dial to select the "Air Crisp" mode.
8. Press the Time button and again turn the dial to set the cooking time to 40 minutes
9. Now push the Temp button and rotate the dial to set the temperature at 330 degrees F.
10. Press "Start/Pause" button to start.
11. When the unit beeps to show that it is preheated, open the lid.
12. Arrange the pan in "Air Fry Basket" and insert in the oven.
13. Place the pan onto a wire rack to cool for about 10 minutes
14. Carefully, invert the bread onto wire rack to cool completely before slicing.
15. Cut the bread into desired-sized slices and serve.

Nutrition:

Calories 384

Fat 23 g

Carbs 39.3 g

Protein 8.9 g

CHAPTER 10:

Deserts

194. Mini cheesecakes

Difficulty: Very Easy

Preparation Time: 15 minutes

Cooking Time: 10 minutes

Servings: 2

Ingredients:

- ¾ cup erythritol
- eggs
- 1 teaspoon vanilla extract
- ½ teaspoon fresh lemon juice
- oz. Cream cheese, softened
- tablespoon sour cream

Directions:

1 In a blender, add the erythritol, eggs, vanilla extract, lemon juice and pulse until smooth.

2 Add the cream cheese and sour cream and pulse until smooth.

3 Place the mixture into 2 (4-inch) spring form pans evenly.

4 Press "power button" of air fry oven and turn the dial to select the "air fry" mode.

5 Press the time button and again turn the dial to set the **Cooking Time:** to 10 minutes.

6 Now push the temp button and rotate the dial to set the temperature at 350 degrees f.

7 Press "start/pause" button to start.

8 When the unit beeps to show that it is preheated, open the lid.

9 Arrange the pans in "air fry basket" and insert in the oven.

10 Place the pans onto a wire rack to cool completely.

11 Refrigerate overnight before serving.

Nutrition:

Calories 886

Total fat 86 g

Saturated fat 52.8 g

Cholesterol 418 mg

Sodium 740 mg

Total carbs 7.2 g

Fiber 0 g

Sugar 1.1 g

Protein 23.1 g

195. Vanilla cheesecake

Difficulty: Very Easy

Preparation Time: 15 minutes

Cooking Time: 14 minutes

Servings: 6

Ingredients:

- 1 cup honey graham cracker crumbs
- tablespoons unsalted butter, softened
- 1 (453.592g). Cream cheese, softened

- ½ cup sugar
- large eggs
- ½ teaspoon vanilla extract

Directions:

1 Line a round baking pan with parchment paper.
2 For crust: in a bowl, add the graham cracker crumbs, and butter.
3 Place the crust into baking dish and press to smooth.
4 Press "power button" of air fry oven and turn the dial to select the "air fry" mode.
5 Press the time button and again turn the dial to set the **Cooking Time:** to 4 minutes.
6 Now push the temp button and rotate the dial to set the temperature at 350 degrees f.
7 Press "start/pause" button to start.
8 When the unit beeps to show that it is preheated, open the lid.
9 Arrange the baking pan of crust in "air fry basket" and insert in the oven.
10 Place the crust aside to cool for about 10 minutes.
11 Meanwhile, in a bowl, add the cream cheese, and sugar and whisk until smooth.
12 Now, place the eggs, one at a time and whisk until mixture becomes creamy.
13 Add the vanilla extract and mix well.
14 Place the cream cheese mixture evenly over the crust.
15 Press "power button" of air fry oven and turn the dial to select the "air fry" mode.
16 Press the time button and again turn the dial to set the **Cooking Time:** to 10 minutes.
17 Now push the temp button and rotate the dial to set the temperature at 350 degrees f.
18 Press "start/pause" button to start.
19 When the unit beeps to show that it is preheated, open the lid.
20 Arrange the baking pan of crust in "air fry basket" and insert in the oven.
21 Place the pan onto a wire rack to cool completely.
22 Refrigerate overnight before serving.

Nutrition:

Calories 470

Total fat 33.9 g

Saturated fat 20.6 g

Cholesterol 155 mg

Sodium 42 mg

Total carbs 34.9 g

Fiber 0.5 g Sugar 22 g

Protein 9.4 g

196. Ricotta cheesecake

Difficulty: Very Easy

Preparation Time: 15 minutes

Cooking Time: 25 minutes

Servings: 8

Ingredients:

- 17.6 oz. Ricotta cheese
- eggs
- ¾ cup sugar
- tablespoons corn starch
- 1 tablespoon fresh lemon juice
- teaspoons vanilla extract
- 1 teaspoon fresh lemon zest, finely grated

Directions:

1 In a large bowl, place all ingredients and mix until well combined.
2 Place the mixture into a baking pan.
3 Press "power button" of air fry oven and turn the dial to select the "air fry" mode. Press the time button and again turn the dial to set the **Cooking Time:** to 25 minutes.
4 Now push the temp button and rotate the dial to set the temperature at 320 degrees f. Press "start/pause" button to start.
5 When the unit beeps to show that it is preheated, open the lid.
6 Arrange the pan in "air fry basket" and insert in the oven.
7 Place the cake pan onto a wire rack to cool completely.
8 Refrigerate overnight before serving.

Nutrition:

Calories 197 Total fat 6.6 g Saturated fat 3.6 g

Cholesterol 81 mg Sodium 102 mg

Total carbs 25.7 g Fiber 0 g Sugar 19.3 g

Protein 9.2 g

197. Pecan pie

Difficulty: Very Easy

Preparation Time: 15 minutes

Cooking Time: 35 minutes

Servings: 5

Ingredients:

- ¾ cup brown sugar
- ¼ cup caster sugar
- 1/3 cup butter, melted
- large eggs
- 1¾ tablespoons flour
- 1 tablespoon milk
- 1 teaspoon vanilla extract
- 1 cup pecan halves
- 1 frozen pie crust, thawed

Directions:

1 In a large bowl, mix the sugars, and butter.
2 Add the eggs and whisk until foamy.
3 Add the flour, milk, and vanilla extract and whisk until well combined.
4 Fold in the pecan halves.
5 Grease a pie pan.
6 Arrange the crust in the bottom of prepared pie pan.
7 Place the pecan mixture over the crust evenly. Press "power button" of air fry oven and turn the dial to select the "air fry" mode.
8 Press the time button and again turn the dial to set the **Cooking Time:** to 22 minutes.
9 Now push the temp button and rotate the dial to set the temperature at 300 degrees f.
10 Press "start/pause" button to start.
11 When the unit beeps to show that it is preheated, open the lid.
12 Arrange the pan in "air fry basket" and insert in the oven.
13 After 22 minutes of cooking, to set the temperature at w85 degrees f for 13 minutes. Place the pie pan onto a wire rack to cool for about 10-15 minutes before serving.

Nutrition:

Calories 501 Total fat 35 g Saturated fat 10.8 g

Cholesterol 107 mg Sodium 187 mg Protein 6.2 g

Total carbs 44.7 g Fiber 2.9 g Sugar 36.7 g

198. Fruity crumble

Difficulty: Very Easy

Preparation Time: 15 minutes

Cooking Time: 20 minutes

Servings: 4

Ingredients:

- ½ lb. (226.8g) Fresh apricots, pitted and cubed
- 1 cup fresh blackberries
- 1/3 cup sugar, divided
- 1 tablespoon fresh lemon juice
- 7/8 cup flour
- Pinch of salt
- 1 tablespoon cold water
- ¼ cup chilled butter, cubed

Directions:

1. Grease a baking pan.
2. In a large bowl, mix well apricots, blackberries, 2 tablespoons of sugar, and lemon juice.
3. Spread apricot mixture into the prepared baking pan.
4. In another bowl, add the flour, remaining sugar, salt, water, and butter and mix until a crumbly mixture form.
5. Spread the flour mixture over apricot mixture evenly.
6. Press "power button" of air fry oven and turn the dial to select the "air fry" mode.
7. Press the time button and again turn the dial to set the **Cooking Time:** to 20 minutes.
8. Now push the temp button and rotate the dial to set the temperature at 390 degrees f.
9. Press "start/pause" button to start.
10. When the unit beeps to show that it is preheated, open the lid.
11. Arrange the pan in "air fry basket" and insert in the oven.
12. Place the pan onto a wire rack to cool for about 10-15 minutes before serving.

Nutrition:

Calories 307

Total fat 12.4 g

Saturated fat 7.4 g

Cholesterol 31 mg

Sodium 123 mg

Total carbs 47.3 g

Fiber 3.8 g

Sugar 23.7 g

Protein 4.2 g

199. Cherry clafoutis

Difficulty: Easy

Preparation Time: 15 minutes

Cooking Time: 25 minutes

Servings: 4

Ingredients:

- 1½ cups fresh cherries, pitted
- tablespoons vodka
- ¼ cup flour
- tablespoons sugar
- Pinch of salt
- ½ cup sour cream
- 1 egg
- 1 tablespoon butter
- ¼ cup powdered sugar

Directions:

1 In a bowl, mix the cherries and vodka.
2 In another bowl, mix the flour, sugar, and salt.
3 Add the sour cream, and egg and mix until a smooth dough form.
4 Grease a cake pan.
5 Place flour mixture evenly into the prepared cake pan.
6 Spread cherry mixture over the dough.
7 Place butter on top in the form of dots.
8 Press "power button" of air fry oven and turn the dial to select the "air fry" mode.
9 Press the time button and again turn the dial to set the **Cooking Time:** to 25 minutes.
10 Now push the temp button and rotate the dial to set the temperature at 355 degrees f.
11 Press "start/pause" button to start.
12 When the unit beeps to show that it is preheated, open the lid.
13 Arrange the pan in "air fry basket" and insert in the oven.
14 Place the pan onto a wire rack to cool for about 10-15 minutes before serving.
15 Now, invert the clafoutis onto a platter and sprinkle with powdered sugar.
16 Cut the clafoutis into desired size slices and serve warm.

Nutrition:

Calories 241

Total fat 10.1 g

Saturated fat 5.9 g

Cholesterol 61 mg

Sodium 90 mg

Total carbs 29 g

Fiber 1.3 g

Sugar 20.6 g

Protein 3.9 g

200. Apple bread pudding

Difficulty: Easy

Preparation Time: 15 minutes

Cooking Time: 44 minutes

Servings: 8

Ingredients:

- For bread pudding:
- 10½ oz. Bread, cubed
- ½ cup apple, peeled, cored and chopped
- ½ cup raisins
- ¼ cup walnuts, chopped
- 1½ cups milk
- ¾ cup water
- tablespoons honey
- teaspoons ground cinnamon
- teaspoons cornstarch
- 1 teaspoon vanilla extract
- For topping:
- 1 1/3 cups plain flour
- 3/5 cup brown sugar
- tablespoons butter

Directions:

1 In a large bowl, mix together the bread, apple, raisins, and walnuts.
2 In another bowl, add the remaining pudding ingredients and mix until well combined.

3. Add the milk mixture into bread mixture and mix until well combined.
4. Refrigerate for about 15 minutes, tossing occasionally.
5. For topping: in a bowl, mix together the flour and sugar.
6. With a pastry cutter, cut in the butter until a crumbly mixture form.
7. Place the mixture into 2 baking pans and spread the topping mixture on top of each.
8. Press "power button" of air fry oven and turn the dial to select the "air fry" mode.
9. Press the time button and again turn the dial to set the **Cooking Time:** to 22 minutes.
10. Now push the temp button and rotate the dial and set the temperature at 355 degrees f.
11. Press "start/pause" button to start.
12. When the unit beeps to show that it is preheated, open the lid.
13. Arrange 1 pan in "air fry basket" and insert in the oven.
14. Place the pan onto a wire rack to cool slightly before serving.
15. Repeat with the remaining pan.
16. Serve warm.

Nutrition:

Calories 432 Total fat 14.8 g

Saturated fat 7.4 g

Cholesterol 30 mg

Sodium 353mg

Total carbs 69.1 g

Fiber 2.8 g

Sugar 32 g

Protein 7.9 g

201. Masala Cashew

Difficulty: Easy

Preparation Time: 25 minutes

Cooking Time: 50 Minutes

Servings: 2

Ingredients

- 2 oz. Greek yogurt
- 1 tbsp mango powder
- 8¾ oz. cashew nuts
- Salt and pepper to taste
- 1 tsp coriander powder
- ½ tsp masala powder
- ½ tsp black pepper powder

Directions:

1. Preheat your Fryer to 240 F.
2. In a bowl, mix all powders. Season with salt and pepper.
3. Add cashews and toss to coat well.
4. Place the cashews in your air fryer's basket and cook for 15 minutes. Serve with a garnish of basil.

Nutrition:

Calories: 202;

Fat: 6;

Fiber: 3;

Carbs: 17;

Protein: 10

202. Donuts pudding

Difficulty: Medium

Preparation Time: 15 minutes

Cooking Time: 1 hour

Servings: 6

Ingredients:

- glazed donuts, cut into small pieces
- ¾ cup frozen sweet cherries
- ½ cup raisins
- ½ cup semi-sweet chocolate baking chips.
- ¼ cup sugar
- 1 teaspoon ground cinnamon
- egg yolks
- 1½ cups whipping cream

Directions:

1 In a large bowl, mix together the donut pieces, cherries, raisins, chocolate chips, sugar, and cinnamon.
2 In another bowl, add the egg yolks, and whipping cream and whisk until well combined.
3 Add the egg yolk mixture into doughnut mixture and mix well.
4 Line a baking dish with a piece of foil.
5 Place donuts mixture into the prepared baking pan.
6 Press "power button" of air fry oven and turn the dial to select the "air fry" mode.
7 Press the time button and again turn the dial to set the **Cooking Time:** to 60 minutes.
8 Now push the temp button and rotate the dial to set the temperature at 360 degrees f.
9 Press "start/pause" button to start.
10 When the unit beeps to show that it is preheated, open the lid.
11 Arrange the pan in "air fry basket" and insert in the oven.
12 Place the pan onto a wire rack to cool for about 10-15 minutes before serving.
13 Serve warm.

Nutrition:

Calories 537

Total fat 28.7 g

Saturated fat 12.2 g

Cholesterol 173 mg

Sodium 194 mg

Total carbs 65.1 g

Fiber 2.3 g

Sugar 32.8 g

Protein 6.5 g

203. Buttery scallops

Difficulty: Medium

Preparation Time: 10 minutes

Cooking Time: 25 minutes

Servings: 8

Ingredients

- lb. (907.185g) Scallops
- tablespoons butter, melted
- tablespoons dry white wine
- 1 tablespoon lemon juice
- 1/2 cup parmesan cheese, grated
- 1 teaspoon salt
- 1/2 teaspoon black pepper
- 1 teaspoon garlic powder
- 1 teaspoon dried parsley
- 1/8 teaspoon cayenne pepper

- 1/4 teaspoon sweet paprika
- tablespoons parsley chopped

Directions:

1 Mix everything in a bowl except scallops.
2 Toss in scallops and mix well to coat them.
3 Spread the scallops with the sauce in a baking tray.
4 Press "power button" of air fry oven and turn the dial to select the "bake" mode.
5 Press the time button and again turn the dial to set the **Cooking Time:** to 25 minutes.
6 Now push the temp button and rotate the dial to set the temperature at 350 degrees f.
7 Once preheated, place the scallop's baking tray in the oven and close its lid.
8 Serve warm.

Nutrition:

Calories 227 Total fat 10.1g

Saturated fat 5.7g Cholesterol 89mg

Sodium 388mg Total carbohydrate 5.6g

Dietary fiber 0.1g Total sugars 0.2g Protein 27.8g

204. Crusted scallops

Difficulty: Medium

Preparation Time: 10 minutes

Cooking Time: 20 minutes

Servings: 4

Ingredients

- 1 1/2 lbs. (680.389g) Bay scallops, rinsed
- garlic cloves, minced
- 1/2 cup panko crumbs
- 1 teaspoon onion powder
- tablespoons butter, melted
- 1/2 teaspoon cayenne pepper
- 1 teaspoon garlic powder
- 1/4 cup parmesan cheese, shredded

Directions:

1 Mix everything in a bowl except scallops.
2 Toss in scallops and mix well to coat them.
3 Spread the scallops with the sauce in a baking tray.
4 Press "power button" of air fry oven and turn the dial to select the "bake" mode.
5 Press the time button and again turn the dial to set the **Cooking Time:** to 20 minutes.
6 Now push the temp button and rotate the dial to set the temperature at 400 degrees f.
7 Once preheated, place the scallop's baking tray in the oven and close its lid.

Nutrition:

Calories 242

Total fat 11.1g

Saturated fat 6.4g

Cholesterol 65mg

Sodium 500mg

Total carbohydrate 11.1g

Dietary fiber 0.7g

Total sugars 0.9g

Protein 23.8g

205. Lobster tails with white wine sauce

Difficulty: Medium

Preparation Time: 10 minutes

Cooking Time: 14 minutes

Servings: 4

Ingredients

- lobster tails, shell cut from the top
- 1/2 onion, quartered
- 1/2 cup butter
- 1/3 cup wine
- 1/4 cup honey
- garlic cloves crushed
- 1 tablespoon lemon juice
- 1 teaspoon salt or to taste
- Cracked pepper to taste
- Lemon slices to serve
- tablespoons fresh chopped parsley

Directions:

1 Place the lobster tails in the oven's baking tray.
2 Whisk rest of the ingredients in a bowl and pour over the lobster tails.
3 Press "power button" of air fry oven and turn the dial to select the "broil" mode.
4 Press the time button and again turn the dial to set the **Cooking Time:** to 14 minutes.
5 Now push the temp button and rotate the dial to set the temperature at 350 degrees f.
6 Once preheated, place the lobster's baking tray in the oven and close its lid.
7 Serve warm.

Nutrition:

Calories 340

Total fat 23.1g

Saturated fat 14.6g

Cholesterol 61mg

Sodium 1249mg

Total carbohydrate 20.4g

Dietary fiber 0.3g

Total sugars 18.1g

Protein 0.7g

206. Broiled lobster tails

Difficulty: Medium

Preparation Time: 10 minutes

Cooking Time: 6 minutes

Servings: 4

Ingredients

- lobster tails, shell cut from the top
- 1/2 cup butter, melted
- 1/2 teaspoon ground paprika
- Salt to taste
- White pepper, to taste
- 1 lemon, juiced

Directions:

1 Place the lobster tails in the oven's baking tray.
2 Whisk rest of the ingredients in a bowl and pour over the lobster tails.
3 Press "power button" of air fry oven and turn the dial to select the "broil" mode.
4 Press the time button and again turn the dial to set the **Cooking Time:** to 6 minutes.

5 Now push the temp button and rotate the dial to set the temperature at 350 degrees f.
6 Once preheated, place the lobster's baking tray in the oven and close its lid.
7 Serve warm.

Nutrition:

Calories 227

Total fat 23.1g

Saturated fat 14.6g

Cholesterol 61mg

Sodium 414mg

Total carbohydrate 0.2g

Dietary fiber 0.1g

Total sugars 0.1g

Protein 20.3g

207. Paprika lobster tail

Difficulty: Medium

Preparation Time: 10 minutes

Cooking Time: 10 minutes

Servings: 4

Ingredients:

- (4 to 6 oz.) lobster tails, shell cut from the top
- 1/8 teaspoon salt
- 1/8 teaspoon black pepper
- 1/8 teaspoon paprika
- tablespoon butter
- 1/2 lemon, cut into wedges
- Chopped parsley for garnish

Directions:

1 Place the lobster tails in the oven's baking tray.
2 Whisk rest of the ingredients in a bowl and pour over the lobster tails.
3 Press "power button" of air fry oven and turn the dial to select the "broil" mode.
4 Press the time button and again turn the dial to set the **Cooking Time:** to 10 minutes.
5 Now push the temp button and rotate the dial to set the temperature at 350 degrees f.
6 Once preheated, place the lobster's baking tray in the oven and close its lid.
7 Serve warm.

Nutrition:

Calories 204 Total fat 12.5g Saturated fat 7.5g

Cholesterol 196mg Sodium 780mg

Total carbohydrate 0.2g Dietary fiber 0.1g

Total sugars 0g Protein 21.7g

208. Lobster tails with lemon butter

Difficulty: Hard

Preparation Time: 10 minutes

Cooking Time: 8 minutes

Servings: 4

Ingredients

- lobster tails, shell cut from the top
- 1 tablespoon fresh parsley, chopped
- garlic cloves, pressed
- 1 teaspoon dijon mustard

- 1/4 teaspoon salt
- 1/8 teaspoon black pepper
- 1 1/2 tablespoon olive oil
- 1 1/2 tablespoon fresh lemon juice
- tablespoon butter, divided

Directions:

1 Place the lobster tails in the oven's baking tray.
2 Whisk rest of the ingredients in a bowl and pour over the lobster tails.
3 Press "power button" of air fry oven and turn the dial to select the "broil" mode.
4 Press the time button and again turn the dial to set the **Cooking Time:** to 8 minutes.
5 Now push the temp button and rotate the dial to set the temperature at 350 degrees f.
6 Once preheated, place the lobster's baking tray in the oven and close its lid.
7 Serve warm.

Nutrition:

Calories 281 Total fat 18.1g Saturated fat 8.4g

Cholesterol 242mg Sodium 950mg

Total carbohydrate 0.8g Dietary fiber 0.1g

Total sugars 0.2g Protein 27.9g

209. Sheet pan seafood bake

Difficulty: Hard

Preparation Time: 10 minutes

Cooking Time: 14 minutes

Servings: 4

Ingredients

- corn ears, husked and diced
- 1 lb. (453.592g) Red potatoes, boiled, diced
- lbs. (907.185g) Clams, scrubbed
- 1 lb. (453.592g) Shrimp, peeled and de-veined
- oz. Sausage, sliced
- 1/2 red onion, sliced
- lobster tails, peeled
- Black pepper to taste
- 1 lemon, cut into wedges
- 1 cup butter
- teaspoons minced garlic
- 1 tablespoon old bay seasoning
- Fresh parsley for garnish

Directions:

1 Toss all the veggies, corn, seafood, oil, and seasoning in a baking tray.
2 Press "power button" of air fry oven and turn the dial to select the "broil" mode.
3 Press the time button and again turn the dial to set the **Cooking Time:** to 14 minutes.
4 Now push the temp button and rotate the dial to set the temperature at 425 degrees f.
5 Once preheated, place the seafood's baking tray in the oven and close its lid.
6 Serve warm.

Nutrition:

Calories 532 Total fat 35.6g

Saturated fat 18.8g Cholesterol 219mg

Sodium 1379mg Total carbohydrate 26.3g

Dietary fiber 2.5g Total sugars 4.4

Protein 28.7g

210. Orange sponge cake

Difficulty: Hard

Preparation Time: 50 minutes

Cooking Time: 14 minutes

Servings: 6

Ingredients

- oz. sugar
- oz. self-rising flour
- oz. butter
- eggs
- 1 tsp baking powder
- 1 tsp vanilla extract
- Zest of 1 orange
- Frosting:
- egg whites
- Juice of 1 orange
- 1 tsp orange food coloring
- Zest of 1 orange
- oz. superfine sugar

Directions:

1 Preheat breville on bake function to 160 f and place all cake ingredients, in a bowl and beat with an electric mixer. Transfer half of the batter into a prepared cake pan; bake for 15 minutes. Repeat the process for the other half of the batter.

2 Meanwhile, prepare the frosting by beating all frosting ingredients together. Spread the frosting mixture on top of one cake. Top with the other cake.

Nutrition:

Calories: 828, Protein: 11.46 g,

Fat: 39.77g, Carbs: 107.89g

211. Apricot crumble with blackberries

Difficulty: Hard

Preparation Time: 30 minutes

Cooking Time: 14 minutes

Servings: 4

Ingredients:

- ½ cups fresh apricots, de-stoned and cubed
- 1 cup fresh blackberries
- ½ cup sugar
- tbsp lemon juice
- 1 cup flour
- Salt as needed
- tbsp butter

Directions:

1 Add the apricot cubes to a bowl and mix with lemon juice, 2 tbsp sugar, and blackberries. Scoop the mixture into a greased dish and spread it evenly. In another bowl, mix flour and remaining sugar.

2 Add 1 tbsp of cold water and butter and keep mixing until you have a crumbly mixture. Preheat breville on bake function to 390 f and place the fruit mixture in the basket. Top with crumb mixture and cook for 20 minutes.

Nutrition:

Calories: 546,

Protein: 7g,

Fat: 5.23g,

Carbs: 102.53g

212. Apple & cinnamon pie

Difficulty: Hard

Preparation Time: 30 minutes

Cooking Time: 14 minutes

Servings: 9

Ingredients:

- apples, diced
- oz. butter, melted
- oz. sugar
- 1 oz. brown sugar
- tsp cinnamon
- 1 egg, beaten
- large puff pastry sheets
- ¼ tsp salt

Directions:

1 Whisk white sugar, brown sugar, cinnamon, salt, and butter, together. Place the apples in a baking dish and coat them with the mixture. Place the baking dish in the toaster oven, and cook for 10 minutes at 350 f on bake function.

2 Meanwhile, roll out the pastry on a floured flat surface, and cut each sheet into 6 equal pieces. Divide the apple filling between the components. Brush the edges of the pastry squares with the egg.

3 Fold them and seal the edges with a fork. Place on a lined baking sheet and cook in the fryer at 350 f for 8 minutes. Flip over, increase the temperature to 390 f, and cook for 2 more minutes.

Nutrition:

Calories: 140,

Protein: 1.28g,

Fat: 6.33g,

Carbs: 21.19g

CHAPTER 11:

Fish and Seafood Recipes

213. Carp Best Homemade Croquette

Difficulty: Very Easy

Preparation Time: 15 minutes

Cooking Time: 25 minutes

Servings: 3

Ingredients:

- 1 lb. Carp filets
- onions chopped
- green chilies-roughly chopped
- 1 ½ tbsp. ginger paste
- 1 ½ tsp garlic paste
- 1 ½ tsp salt
- tsp lemon juice
- tsp garam masala
- tbsp. chopped coriander
- tbsp. cream
- tbsp. coriander powder
- tbsp. fresh mint chopped
- tbsp. chopped capsicum
- eggs
- ½ tbsp. white sesame seeds

Directions:

1 Take all the ingredients mentioned under the first heading and mix them in a bowl. Grind them thoroughly to make a smooth paste. Take the eggs in a different bowl and beat them. Add a pinch of salt and leave them aside. Mold the fish mixture into small balls and flatten them into round and flat Best Homemade Croquettes. Dip these Best Homemade Croquettes in the egg and salt mixture and then in the mixture of breadcrumbs and sesame seeds.

2 Leave these Best Homemade Croquettes in the fridge for an hour or so to set. Pre heat the Breville smart oven at 160 degrees Fahrenheit for around 5 minutes. Place the Best Homemade Croquettes in the basket and let them cook for another 25 minutes at the same temperature. Turn the Best Homemade Croquettes over in between the cooking process to get a uniform cook. Serve the Best Homemade Croquettes with mint sauce.

Nutrition:

Calories: 209; Fat: 4g; Protein: 49g; Sugar: 1g

214. Shrimp Momo's Recipe

Difficulty: Very Easy

Preparation Time: 10 minutes

Cooking Time: 20 minutes

Servings: 7

Ingredients:

- 1 ½ cup all-purpose flour
- ½ tsp. salt
- tbsp. water
- For filling:
- cups minced shrimp
- tbsp. oil
- tsp. ginger-garlic paste
- tsp. soya sauce
- tsp. vinegar

Directions:

1 Squeeze out the dough and cover it with plastic wrap and set it aside. Then cook the ingredients for the filling and try to make sure the shrimp are well coated with the sauce. Roll up the dough and cut it into squares. Place the filling in the center.

2 Now, roll the dough to cover the filling and bring the edges together. Preheat the Breville Smart Oven to 200 ° F for 5 minutes. Place the wontons in the pan and close it. Let them cook at the equal temperature for another 20 minutes. Recommended sides are chili sauce or ketchup.

Nutrition:

Calories: 103;

Fat: 0g;

Protein: 34g;

Sugar: 11

215. Salmon fries

Difficulty: Very Easy

Preparation Time: 5 minutes

Cooking Time: 15 minutes

Servings: 3

Ingredients:

- 1 lb. boneless salmon filets
- cup dry breadcrumbs
- tsp. oregano
- tsp. red chili flakes
- 1 ½ tbsp. ginger-garlic paste
- tbsp. lemon juice
- tsp. salt
- 1 tsp. pepper powder
- 1 tsp. red chili powder
- tbsp. corn flour
- eggs

Directions:

1 Mix each and every ingredients for the marinade and put the salmon fillets and leave to rest overnight. Mix the toast, oregano, and red chili flakes well and place the marinated oregano fingers in this mixture. Cover with cling film and leave until served.

2 Preheat the Breville smart oven to 160 degrees Fahrenheit for 5 minutes.

3 Put the oregano fingers in the pan and close it. Let them cook at the equal temperature for another 15 minutes or so. Toss the oregano fingers well so that they are well cooked.

Nutrition:

Calories: 300;

Fat: 3g;

Protein: 16g;

Sugar: 2

216. Oyster Club Sandwich

Difficulty: Very Easy

Preparation Time: 10 minutes

Cooking Time: 15 minutes

Servings: 4

Ingredients:

2 slices of white bread

1 tbsp. softened butter

½ lb. shelled oyster

1 small capsicum

For Barbeque Sauce:

¼ tbsp. Worcestershire sauce

½ tsp. olive oil

½ flake garlic crushed

¼ cup chopped onion

¼ tsp. mustard powder

1 tbsp. tomato ketchup

½ tbsp. sugar

¼ tbsp. red chili sauce

½ cup water.

Salt and black pepper to taste

Directions:

Remove the edges of the slice bread. Now cut the slices horizontally. Cook the ingredients for the sauce and wait till it thickens. Now, add the oyster to the sauce and stir till it obtains the flavors.

Roast the capsicum and peel the skin off. Cut the capsicum into slices. Mix all ingredients together and apply it to the bread slices. Pre-heat the Breville smart oven for 5 minutes at 300 Fahrenheit. Open the basket of the Fryer and place the prepared Classic Sandwiches in it such that no two Classic Sandwiches are touching each other. Now keep the fryer at 250 degrees for around 15 minutes.

Turn the Classic Sandwiches in between the cooking process to cook both slices. Serve the Classic Sandwiches with tomato ketchup or mint sauce.

Nutrition:

Calories: 407; Fat: 10g; Protein: 31g; Sugar: 11

217. Cheese Carp Fries

Difficulty: Very Easy

Preparation Time: 15 minutes

Cooking Time: 25 minutes

Servings: 4

Ingredients:

- 1 lb. carp Oregano Fingers
- Ingredients for the marinade:
- 1 tbsp. olive oil

- 1 tsp. mixed herbs
- ½ tsp. red chili flakes
- A pinch of salt to taste
- 1 tbsp. lemon juice
- For the garnish:
- 1 cup melted cheddar cheese

Directions:

1. Take all the ingredients mentioned in the heading "For the marinade" and mix well. Cook the oregano fingers and dip them in the marinade.
2. Preheat the Breville smart oven for about 5 minutes at 300 Fahrenheit. Take the basket out of the fryer and place the tent in it. Close the basket. Now keep the fryer at 220 Fahrenheit for 20 to 25 minutes.
3. Between the processes, toss the potatoes two or three times so they are cooked through. Towards the rare end of the cooking process (the last 2 minutes or so), sprinkle the melted cheddar cheese over the potatoes and serve hot.

Nutrition:

Calories: 502; Fat: 22g; Protein: 40g; Sugar: 14

218. Seafood Pizza

Difficulty: Very Easy

Preparation Time: 10 minutes

Cooking Time: 22 minutes

Servings: 4

Ingredients:

- One pizza base
- Grated pizza cheese (mozzarella cheese preferably) for topping
- Some pizza topping sauce
- Use cooking oil for brushing and topping purposes
- Ingredients for topping:
- onions chopped
- cups mixed seafood
- capsicums chopped
- tomatoes that have been deseeded and chopped
- 1 tbsp. (optional) mushrooms/corns
- tsp. pizza seasoning
- Some cottage cheese that has been cut into small cubes (optional)

Directions:

1 Put the pizza base in a pre-heated Breville smart oven for around 5 minutes. (Pre heated to 340 Fahrenheit). Take out the base. Pour some pizza sauce on top of the base at the center. Using a spoon spread the sauce over the base making sure that you leave some gap around the circumference. Grate some mozzarella cheese and sprinkle it over the sauce layer. Take all the vegetables and the seafood and mix them in a bowl. Add some oil and seasoning.

2 Also add some salt and pepper according to taste. Mix them properly. Put this topping over the layer of cheese on the pizza. Now sprinkle some more grated cheese and pizza seasoning on top of this layer. Pre

heat the Breville smart oven at 250 Fahrenheit for around 5 minutes.

3 Open the fry basket and place the pizza inside. Close the basket and keep the fryer at 170 degrees for another 10 minutes. If you feel that it is undercooked you may put it at the same temperature for another 2 minutes or so.

Nutrition:

Calories: 116;

Fat: 23g;

Protein: 29g;

Sugar: 1

219. Lobster Grandma's Easy to Cook Wontons

Difficulty: Very Easy

Preparation Time: 10 minutes

Cooking Time: 20 minutes

Servings: 4

Ingredients:

- 1 ½ cup all-purpose flour
- ½ tsp. salt
- tbsp. water
- For filling:
- cups minced lobster
- tbsp. oil
- tsp. ginger-garlic paste
- tsp. soya sauce
- tsp. vinegar

Directions:

1 Squeeze out the dough and cover it with plastic wrap and set it aside. Then cook the ingredients for the filling and try to make sure the lobster is well coated with the sauce.

2 Roll out the dough and place the filling in the center. Now, roll the dough to cover the filling and bring the edges together.

3 Preheat the Breville Smart Oven to 200 ° F for 5 minutes. Place the wontons in the pan and close it. Let them cook at the equal temperature for another 20 minutes. Recommended sides are chili sauce or ketchup.

Nutrition:

Calories: 600;

Fat: 13g;

Protein: 21g;

Sugar: 9

220. Cilantro-Lime Fried Shrimp

Difficulty: Very Easy

Preparation Time: 10 minutes

Cooking Time: 10 minutes

Servings: 4

Ingredients:

- ½ cup chopped fresh cilantro
- Juice of 1 lime
- 1 pound of raw shrimp, deveined and peeled with tails on or off

- 1 egg
- ½ cup all-purpose flour
- ¾ cup bread crumbs
- Salt
- Pepper
- Cooking oil
- ½ cup cocktail sauce (optional)

Directions:

1 Place the shrimp in a plastic bag. Add the cilantro and lime juice. Seal the bag. Shake to combine. Marinate in the refrigerator for 30 minutes.

2 In a small bowl, beat the egg. In another small bowl, place the flour. Place the crumbs of bread in a third small bowl, and season with salt and pepper to taste.

3 Spray cooking oil to the air fryer basket.

4 Remove the shrimp from the plastic bag. Wet each in the flour, then the egg, and then the bread crumbs.

5 Place the shrimp in the air fryer. It is okay to stack them. Spray the shrimp with cooking oil. Cook for 4 minutes.

6 Open the air fryer and flip the shrimp. I recommend scanning individually instead of shaking to keep the breading intact. Cook for another 4 minutes, or until crisp.

7 Cool before serving. Serve with cocktail sauce if desired.

8 Substitution tip: You can reduce the number of calories and fat in this recipe by substituting an egg white for the whole egg.

9 Preparation tip: If using frozen shrimp, place the shrimp in a large bowl of cold water to thaw. Let the shrimp to soak for 15 minutes.

Nutrition:

Calories: 254

Total fat: 4g

Saturated fat: 1g

Cholesterol: 221mg

Sodium: 334mg

Carbohydrates: 27g

Fiber: 1g

Protein: 29g

221. Salmon Croquettes

Difficulty: Very Easy

Preparation Time: 5 minutes

Cooking Time: 15 minutes

Servings: 6

Ingredients:

- 1 (14.75-ounce) can Alaskan pink salmon, drained and bones removed
- 1 egg, beaten
- ½ cup bread crumbs
- scallions, diced
- 1 teaspoon garlic powder
- Salt
- Pepper
- Cooking oil

Directions:

1 In a large bowl, combine the salmon, beaten egg, bread crumbs, and scallions. Season with the garlic powder and salt and pepper to taste.

2 Form the mixture into 6 patties.

3 Place the croquettes in the air fryer. It is okay to stack them. Spray the croquettes with cooking oil. Cook for 7 minutes.

4 Open the air fryer and flip the patties. Cook for an additional 3 to 4 minutes, or until golden brown.

5 Serve.

Nutrition:

Calories: 142

Total fat: 6g

Saturated fat: 1g

Cholesterol: 58mg

Sodium: 135mg

Carbohydrates: 7g

Fiber: 1g

Protein: 16g

222. Beer-Battered Fish and Chips

Difficulty: Very Easy

Preparation Time: 5 minutes

Cooking Time: 30 minutes

Servings: 4

Ingredients:

- eggs
- 1 cup malty beer, such as Pabst Blue Ribbon
- 1 cup all-purpose flour
- ½ cup cornstarch
- 1 teaspoon garlic powder
- Salt
- Pepper
- Cooking oil
- (4-ounce) cod fillets

Directions:

1 Beat the eggs with the beer. In another medium bowl, combine the flour and cornstarch, and season with the garlic powder and salt and pepper to taste.

2 Spray cooking oil to the air fryer basket.

3 Dip each cod fillet in the flour and cornstarch mixture and then in the egg and beer mixture. Dip the cod in the flour and cornstarch a second time.

4 Place the cod in the air fryer. Do not stack. Cook in batches. Spray with cooking oil. Cook for 8 minutes.

5 Open the air fryer and flip the cod. Cook for an additional 7 minutes.

6 Remove the cooked cod from the air fryer, then repeat steps 4 and 5 for the remaining fillets.

7 Serve with Classic French Fries or prepare air-fried frozen fries. Frozen fries will need to be cooked for 18 to 20 minutes at 400°F.

8 Cool before serving.

Nutrition:

Calories: 325 Total fat: 4g

Saturated fat: 1g Cholesterol: 137mg

Sodium: 144mg Carbohydrates: 41g Fiber: 1g

Protein: 26g

223. Firecracker Shrimp

Difficulty: Very Easy

Preparation Time: 10 minutes

Cooking Time: 10 minutes

Servings: 4

Ingredients:

- For the shrimp
- 1-pound raw shrimp, peeled and deveined
- Salt
- Pepper
- 1 egg
- ½ cup all-purpose flour
- ¾ cup panko bread crumbs
- Cooking oil
- For the firecracker sauce
- 1/3 cup sour cream
- tablespoons Sriracha
- ¼ cup sweet chili sauce

Directions:

1 To make the shrimp

2 Add the shrimp with pepper and salt to taste.

3 In a small bowl, beat the egg.

4 In another small bowl, place the flour. In another small bowl, add the panko bread crumbs.

5 Spray cooking oil to the air fryer basket.

6 Dip the shrimp in the flour, then the egg, and then the bread crumbs.

7 Place the shrimp in the fryer basket. It is okay to stack them. Spray the shrimp with cooking oil. Cook for 4 minutes.

8 Open the air fryer and flip the shrimp. I recommend scanning individually instead of shaking to keep the breading intact.

9 Cook for another 4 minutes or until crisp.

10 To make the firecracker sauce

11 While the shrimp is cooking, make the firecracker sauce: In a small bowl, combine the sour cream, Sriracha, and sweet chili sauce. Mix well.

12 Serve with the shrimp.

13 Substitution tip: In place of sour cream, use nonfat plain Greek yogurt. This saves calories and fat while providing 5.5 grams additional protein.

Nutrition:

Calories: 266 Total fat: 6g

Saturated fat: 3g Cholesterol: 229mg

Sodium: 393mg Carbohydrates: 23g Fiber: 1g

Protein: 27g

224. Crab Cakes

Difficulty: Easy

Preparation Time: 5 minutes

Cooking Time: 10 minutes

Servings: 4

Ingredients:

- ounces jumbo lump crabmeat
- 1 tablespoon Old Bay Seasoning
- 1/3 cup bread crumbs
- ¼ cup diced red bell pepper
- ¼ cup diced green bell pepper
- 1 egg
- ¼ cup mayonnaise
- Juice of ½ lemon
- 1 teaspoon flour
- Cooking oil

Directions:

1 In a bowl, combine the crab meat, Old Bay Seasoning, bread crumbs, red bell pepper, green bell pepper, egg, mayo, and lemon juice. Mix gently to combine. Form the mixture into ,4 patties. Sprinkle ¼ teaspoon of flour on top of each cake.

2 Place the crab cakes in the air fryer. Spray them with cooking oil. Cook for 10 minutes. Serve.

3 Ingredient tip: You can make your own crab seasoning using ¼ teaspoon of each of the following: celery salt, black pepper, red pepper flakes, and paprika.

Nutrition:

Calories: 176

Total fat: 8g

Saturated fat: 1g

Cholesterol: 101mg

Sodium: 826mg

Carbohydrates: 12g

Fiber: 1g

Protein: 15g

225. Coconut Shrimp

Difficulty: Easy

Preparation Time: 10 minutes

Cooking Time: 10 minutes

Servings: 4

Ingredients:

- 1-pound raw shrimp, peeled and deveined
- 1 egg
- ¼ cup all-purpose flour
- 1/3 cup shredded unsweetened coconut
- ¼ cup panko bread crumbs
- Salt
- Pepper
- Cooking oil

Directions:

1 Dry the shrimp with paper towels.

2 In a small bowl, beat the egg. In another small bowl, place the flour. In a third small bowl, combine the coconut and panko bread crumbs,

and season with salt and pepper to taste. Mix well.

3 Spray cooking oil to the air fryer basket.

4 Dip the shrimp in the flour, then the egg, and then the coconut and bread crumb mixture.

5 Place the shrimp in the air fryer. It is okay to stack them. Cook for 4 minutes.

6 Open the air fryer and flip the shrimp. I recommend flipping individually instead of shaking, which keeps the breading intact. Cook for another 4 minutes or until crisp.

7 Cool before serving.

Nutrition:

Calories: 182 Total fat: 6g

Saturated fat: 3g Cholesterol: 246mg

Sodium: 780mg Carbohydrates: 8g

Fiber: 1g Protein: 24g

226. Lemon-Pepper Tilapia with Garlic Aioli

Difficulty: Easy

Preparation Time: 5 minutes

Cooking Time: 15 minutes

Servings: 4

Ingredients:

- For the tilapia
- tilapia fillets
- 1 tablespoon extra-virgin olive oil
- 1 teaspoon paprika
- 1 teaspoon garlic powder
- 1 teaspoon dried basil
- Lemon-pepper seasoning (such as McCormick Perfect Pinch Lemon & Pepper Seasoning)
- For the garlic aioli
- garlic cloves, minced
- 1 tablespoon mayonnaise
- 1 teaspoon extra-virgin olive oil
- Juice of ½ lemon
- Salt
- Pepper

Directions:

1 To make the tilapia

2 Coat the fish with the olive oil. Season with the paprika, garlic powder, dried basil, and lemon-pepper seasoning.

3 Place the fish in the air fryer. It is okay to stack the fish. Cook for 8 minutes.

4 Open the fryer and flip the fish. Cook for an additional 7 minutes.

5 To make the garlic aioli

6 In a bowl, put together the garlic, mayonnaise, olive oil, lemon juice, and salt and pepper to taste. Whisk well to combine.

7 Serve alongside the fish.

8 Variation tip: This recipe can be gluten-free by using gluten-free mayonnaise; be sure to check the label.

9 Ingredient tip: You can make your lemon-pepper seasoning using the juice of ½ lemon and pepper to taste.

10 Preparation tip: If using frozen tilapia, the best way to thaw it is in a covered bowl in the refrigerator, overnight. You can keep the fish in a sealed plastic bag and submerge the bag in cold water for 15 minutes or till thawed.

Nutrition:

Calories: 155

Total fat: 7g

Saturated fat: 1g

Cholesterol: 56mg

Sodium: 107mg

Carbohydrates: 2g

Fiber: 0g

Protein: 21g

227. Blackened Shrimp

Difficulty: Easy

Preparation Time: 5 minutes

Cooking Time: 10 minutes

Servings: 4

Ingredients:

- 1-pound raw shrimp, peeled and deveined
- 1 teaspoon paprika
- ½ teaspoon dried oregano
- ½ teaspoon cayenne pepper
- Juice of ½ lemon
- Salt
- Pepper
- Cooking oil

Directions:

1 Put the shrimp in a sealable plastic bag then add the paprika, oregano, cayenne pepper, lemon juice, and salt and pepper to taste. Seal the bag. Shake well to combine.

2 Spray a grill pan or the air fryer basket with cooking oil.

3 Place the shrimp in the air fryer. It is okay to stack the shrimp. Cook for 4 minutes.

4 Open the air fryer then after that, shake the basket. Heat for an additional of 3 to 4 minutes, or till the shrimp has blackened.

5 Cool before serving.

6 Variation tip: This shrimp is delicious over a green salad with avocado. Dress it with a simple cilantro-lime vinaigrette made from chopped fresh cilantro, lime juice, and olive oil.

Nutrition:

Calories: 101

Total fat: 2g

Saturated fat: 2g

Cholesterol: 168mg

Sodium: 759mg

Carbohydrates: 0g

Fiber: 0g

Protein: 21g

228. Fried Catfish Nuggets

Difficulty: Easy

Preparation Time: 5 minutes

Cooking Time: 40 minutes

Servings: 4

Ingredients:

- 1-pound catfish fillets, cut into 1-inch chunks
- ½ cup seasoned fish fry breading mix (such as Louisiana Fish Fry)
- Cooking oil

Directions:

1. Rinse and thoroughly dry the catfish. Pour the seasoned fish fry breading mix into a sealable plastic bag and add the catfish. (You may need to use two bags depending on the size of your nuggets.) Seal the bag and shake to coat the fish with breading evenly.
2. Spray cooking oil to the air fryer basket.
3. Transfer the catfish nuggets to the air fryer. Do not overcrowd the basket. You may need to cook the nuggets in two batches. Spray the clumps with cooking oil. Cook for 10 minutes.
4. Open the air fryer then after that, shake the basket. Cook for an additional of 8 to 10 minutes, or till the fish is crisp.
5. If necessary, remove the cooked catfish nuggets from the air fryer, repeat steps 3 and 4 for the remaining fish.
6. Cool before serving.
7. Ingredient tip: You may be able to purchase catfish nuggets at your grocery store's fish counter. It's worth asking!
8. Cooking tip: Open the air fryer and check in on the fish a few times throughout the cooking process. When the fish has turned golden brown on both sides, it has finished cooking.

Nutrition:

Calories: 183

Total fat: 9g

Saturated fat: 2g

Cholesterol: 56mg

Sodium: 199mg

Carbohydrates: 5g

Fiber: 0g

Protein: 19g

229. Cornmeal Shrimp Po'boy

Difficulty: Medium

Preparation Time: 10 minutes

Cooking Time: 10 minutes

Servings: 4

Ingredients:

- For the shrimp
- 1-pound shrimp, peeled and deveined
- 1 egg
- ½ cup flour
- ¾ cup cornmeal
- Salt

- Pepper
- Cooking oil
- For the remoulade
- ½ cup mayonnaise
- 1 teaspoon mustard (I use Dijon)
- 1 teaspoon Worcestershire
- 1 teaspoon minced garlic
- Juice of ½ lemon
- 1 teaspoon Sriracha
- ½ teaspoon Creole seasoning
- For the po'boys
- rolls
- cups shredded lettuce
- slices tomato

Directions:

1 To make the shrimp

2 Dry the shrimp with paper towels.

3 In a small bowl, beat the egg. In another small bowl, place the flour. Place the cornmeal in a third small bowl, and season with salt and pepper to taste.

4 Spray cooking oil to the air fryer basket.

5 Dip the shrimp in the flour, then the egg, and then the cornmeal.

6 Place the shrimp in the air fryer. Cook for 4 minutes. Open the basket and flip the shrimp. Cook for another 4 minutes, or till crisp.

7 To make the remoulade

8 While the shrimp is cooking, in a small bowl, combine the mayonnaise, mustard, Worcestershire, garlic, lemon juice, Sriracha, and Creole seasoning. Mix well.

9 To make the po'boys

10 Split the rolls and spread them with the remoulade.

11 Let the shrimp cool slightly before assembling the po'boys.

12 Fill each roll with a quarter of the shrimp, ½ cup of shredded lettuce, and 2 slices of tomato. Serve.

Nutrition:

Calories: 483

Total fat: 15g

Saturated fat: 2g

Cholesterol: 229mg

Sodium: 690mg

Carbohydrates: 58g

Fiber: 6g

Protein: 32g

230. Spicy Shrimp Kebab

Difficulty: Medium

Preparation Time: 25 minutes

Cooking Time: 20 minutes

Servings: 4

Ingredients:

- 1 ½ pounds jumbo shrimp, cleaned, shelled and deveined
- 1-pound cherry tomatoes

- tablespoons butter, melted
- 1 tablespoons sriracha sauce
- Sea salt and ground black pepper
- 1 2 teaspoon dried oregano
- 1 2 teaspoon dried basil
- 1 teaspoon dried parsley flakes
- 1 2 teaspoon marjoram
- 1 2 teaspoon mustard seeds

Directions:

1 Toss all elements in a mixing bowl until the shrimp and tomatoes are covered on all sides.

2 Let the wooden skewers be soaked in water for 15 minutes.

3 Thread the jumbo shrimp and cherry tomatoes onto skewers. Cook in the preheated air fryer at a temperature of 400 degrees f for 5 minutes, working with batches.

Nutrition:

247 Calories 8.4g Fat 6g Carbohydrates

36.4g Protein 3.5g Sugars 1.8g Fiber

231. Crumbed Fish Fillets with Tarragon

Difficulty: Medium

Preparation Time: 25 minutes

Cooking Time: 20 minutes

Servings: 4

Ingredients:

- eggs, beaten
- 1 2 teaspoon tarragon
- fish fillets, halved
- tablespoons dry white wine
- 1 3 cup parmesan cheese, grated
- 1 teaspoon seasoned salt
- 1 3 teaspoon mixed peppercorns
- 1 2 teaspoon fennel seed

Directions:

1 Add the parmesan cheese, salt, peppercorns, fennel seeds, and tarragon to your food processor; blitz for about 20 seconds.

2 Drizzle fish fillets with dry white wine. Dump the egg into a shallow dish.

3 Now, coat the fish fillets with the beaten egg on all sides; then, coat them with the seasoned cracker mix.

4 Air-fry at 345 degrees f for about 17 minutes.

Nutrition:

305 calories 17.7g fat 6.3g Carbohydrates

27.2g protein 0.3g sugars 0.1g fiber

232. Smoked and Creamed White Fish

Difficulty: Medium

Preparation Time: 20 minutes

Cooking Time: 15 minutes

Servings: 4

Ingredients:

- 1/2 tablespoon yogurt

- 1/3 cup spring garlic, finely chopped
- Fresh chopped chives, for garnish
- eggs, beaten
- 1/2 teaspoon dried dill weed
- 1 teaspoon dried rosemary
- 1/3 cup scallions, chopped
- / 3 cup smoked white fish, chopped
- 1/½ tablespoons crème fraiche
- 1 teaspoon kosher salt
- 1 teaspoon dried marjoram
- 1/3 teaspoon ground black pepper, or more to taste
- Cooking spray

Directions:

1 Firstly, spritz four oven safe ramekins with cooking spray. Then, divide smoked whitefish, spring garlic, and scallions among greased ramekins.

2 Crack an egg into each ramekin; add the crème, yogurt and all seasonings.

3 Now, air-fry approximately 13 minutes at 355 degrees f. Taste for doneness and eat warm garnished with fresh chives.

Nutrition:

249 Calories

22.1g Fat

7.6g Carbohydrates

5.3g Protein

3.1g Sugars

0.7g Fiber

233. Parmesan and Paprika Baked Tilapia

Difficulty: Medium

Preparation Time: 20 minutes

Cooking Time: 15 minutes

Servings: 6

Ingredients:

- 1 cup parmesan cheese, grated
- 1 teaspoon paprika
- 1 teaspoon dried dill weed
- pounds tilapia fillets
- 1 3 cup mayonnaise
- 1 2 tablespoon lime juice
- Salt and ground black pepper, to taste

Directions:

1 Mix the mayonnaise, parmesan, paprika, salt, black pepper, and dill weed until everything is thoroughly combined.

2 Then, drizzle tilapia fillets with the lime juice.

3 Cover each fish fillet with parmesan mayo mixture; roll them in parmesan paprika mixture. Bake to your fryer at 335 for about 10 minutes. Serve and eat warm.

Nutrition:

294 calories 16.1g fat 2.7g Carbohydrates

35.9g protein 0.1g sugars 0.2g fiber

234. Tangy Cod Fillets

Difficulty: Medium

Preparation Time: 20 minutes

Cooking Time: 15 minutes

Servings: 2

Ingredients:

- 1 ½ tablespoons sesame oil
- 1 2 heaping teaspoon dried parsley flakes
- 1 3 teaspoon fresh lemon zest, finely grated
- medium-sized cod fillets
- 1 teaspoon sea salt flakes
- A pinch of salt and pepper
- 1 3 teaspoon ground black pepper, or more to savor
- 1 2 tablespoon fresh lemon juice

Directions:

1 Set the air fryer to cook at 375 degrees f. Season each cod fillet with sea salt flakes, black pepper and dried parsley flakes. Now, drizzle them with sesame oil.

2 Place the seasoned cod fillets in a single layer at the bottom of the cooking basket; air-fry approximately 10 minutes. While the fillets are cooking, prepare the sauce by mixing the other ingredients. Serve cod fillets on four individual plates garnished with the creamy citrus sauce.

Nutrition:

291 calories 11.1g fat 2.7g Carbohydrates

41.6g protein 1.2g sugars 0.5g fiber

235. Fish and Cauliflower Cakes

Difficulty: Medium

Preparation Time: 2 hours 20 minutes

Cooking Time: 13 minutes

Servings: 4

Ingredients:

- 1 2-pound cauliflower florets
- 1 2 teaspoon English mustard
- tablespoons butter, room temperature
- 1 2 tablespoon cilantro, minced
- tablespoons sour cream
- ½ cups cooked white fish
- Salt and freshly cracked black pepper, to savor

Directions:

1 Boil the cauliflower until tender. Then, purée the cauliflower in your blender. Transfer to a mixing dish.

2 Now, stir in the fish, cilantro, salt, and black pepper.

3 Add the sour cream, English mustard, and butter; mix until everything's well incorporated. Using your hands, shape into patties.

4 Place inside the refrigerator for around two hours. Cook in your fryer for 13 minutes at 395 degrees f. Serve with some extra English mustard.

Nutrition:

285 calories 15.1g fat 4.3g Carbohydrates

31.1g protein 1.6g sugars 1.3g fiber

CHAPTER 12:

Poultry Recipes

236. Honey and Wine Chicken Breasts

Difficulty: Very Easy

Preparation Time: 5 Minutes

Cooking Time: 15 Minutes

Servings: 4

Ingredients:

- chicken breasts, rinsed and halved
- 1 tablespoon melted butter
- A pinch of salt and 1/2 tsp freshly ground pepper to taste
- 3/4 teaspoon sea salt, or to taste
- 1 teaspoon paprika
- 1 teaspoon dried rosemary
- tablespoons dry white wine
- 1 tablespoon honey

Directions:

1 Preparing the Ingredients. Firstly, pat the chicken breasts dry. Lightly coat them with the melted butter.

2 Then, add the remaining ingredients.

3 Air Frying. Transfer them to the air fryer rack/basket; bake about 15 minutes at 330 degrees F. Serve warm and enjoy

Nutrition:

Calories: 189;

Fat: 14g;

Protein: 11g;

Sugar: 1

237. Crispy Honey Garlic Chicken Wings

Difficulty: Very Easy

Preparation Time: 10 Minutes

Cooking Time: 25 Minutes

Servings: 8

Ingredients:

- 1/8 C. water
- ½ tsp. salt
- tbsp. minced garlic
- ¼ C. vegan butter
- ¼ C. raw honey
- ¾ C. almond flour
- chicken wings

Directions:

1 Preparing the Ingredients. Rinse off and dry chicken wings well.

2 Spray air fryer rack/basket with olive oil.

3 Coat chicken wings with almond flour and add coated wings to the Air fryer oven.

4 Air Frying. Set temperature to 380°F, and set time to 25 minutes. Cook shaking every 5 minutes.

5 When the timer goes off, cook 5-10 minutes at 400 degrees till skin becomes crispy and dry.

6 As chicken cooks, melt butter in a saucepan and add garlic. Sauté garlic 5 minutes. Add salt and honey, simmering 20 minutes. Make sure to stir every so often, so the sauce does not burn. Add a bit of water after 15 minutes to ensure sauce does not harden.

7 Take out chicken wings from air fryer and coat in sauce. Enjoy!

Nutrition:

Calories: 435;

Fat: 19g;

Protein: 31g;

Sugar: 6

238. Lemon-Pepper Chicken Wings

Difficulty: Very Easy

Preparation Time: 10 Minutes

Cooking Time: 20 Minutes

Servings: 4

Ingredients:

- whole chicken wings
- Juice of ½ lemon
- ½ teaspoon garlic powder
- 1 teaspoon onion powder
- Salt
- Pepper
- ¼ cup low-fat buttermilk
- ½ cup all-purpose flour
- Cooking oil

Directions:

1 Preparing the Ingredients. Place the wings in a sealed plastic bag. Drizzle the wings with the lemon juice. Season the wings with the garlic powder, onion powder, and salt and pepper to taste.

2 Seal the bag. Shake thoroughly to combine the seasonings and coat the wings.

3 Pour the buttermilk and the flour into separate bowls large enough to dip the wings.

4 Spray the Oven rack/basket with cooking oil.

5 One at a time, dip the wings in the buttermilk and then the flour.

6 Air Frying. Place the wings in the Oven rack/basket. It is okay to stack them on top of each other. Spray the wings with cooking oil, being sure to spray the bottom layer. Place the tray rack on the middle-shelf of the Air fryer oven. Set temperature to 360°F and cook for 5 minutes.

7 Remove the basket and shake it to ensure all of the pieces will cook fully.

8 Return the basket to the Air fryer oven and continue to cook the chicken. Repeat shaking every 5 minutes until a total of 20 minutes has passed.

9 Cool before serving.

Nutrition:

Calories: 347;

Fat: 12g;

Protein: 46g;

Fiber: 1g

239. Cheesy Chicken in Leek-Tomato Sauce

Difficulty: Very Easy

Preparation Time: 10 Minutes

Cooking Time: 20 Minutes

Servings: 4

Ingredients:

- Large-sized chicken breasts, cut in half lengthwise
- Salt and ground black pepper, to taste
- Ounces cheddar cheese, cut into sticks
- 1 tablespoon sesame oil
- 1 cup leeks, chopped
- cloves garlic, minced
- 2/3 cup roasted vegetable stock
- 2/3 cup tomato puree
- 1 teaspoon dried rosemary
- 1 teaspoon dried thyme

Directions:

1. Preparing the Ingredients. Firstly, season chicken breasts with the salt and black pepper; place a piece of Cheddar cheese in the middle. Then, tie it using a kitchen string; drizzle with sesame oil and reserve.
2. Add the leeks and garlic to the oven safe bowl.
3. Air Frying. Cook in the Air fryer oven at 390 degrees F for 5 minutes or until tender.
4. Add the reserved chicken. Throw in the other ingredients and cook for 12 to 13 minutes more or 4. Until the chicken is done. Enjoy!

240. Mexican Chicken Burgers

Difficulty: Easy

Preparation Time: 10 Minutes

Cooking Time: 10 Minutes

Servings: 6

Ingredients:

- 1 jalapeno pepper
- 1 tsp. cayenne pepper
- 1 tbsp. mustard powder
- 1 tbsp. oregano
- 1 tbsp. thyme
- tbsp. smoked paprika
- 1 beaten egg
- 1 small head of cauliflower
- chicken breasts

Directions:

1 Preparing the Ingredients. Ensure your Air fryer oven is preheated to 350 degrees.

2 Add seasonings to a blender. Slice cauliflower into florets and add to blender.

3 Pulse till mixture resembles that of breadcrumbs.

4 Take out ¾ of cauliflower mixture and add to a bowl. Set to the side. In another bowl, beat your egg and set to the side.

5 Remove skin and bones from chicken breasts and add to blender with remaining cauliflower mixture. Season with pepper and salt.

6 Take out mixture and form into burger shapes. Roll each patty in cauliflower crumbs, then the egg, and back into crumbs again.

7 Air Frying. Place coated patties into the Air fryer oven. Set temperature to 350°F, and set time to 10 minutes.

8 Flip over at 10-minute mark. They are done when crispy!

Nutrition:

Calories: 234;

Fat: 18g;

Protein: 24g;

Sugar: 1g

241. Minty Chicken-Fried Pork Chops

Difficulty: Easy

Preparation Time: 10 Minutes

Cooking Time: 30 Minutes

Servings: 6

Ingredients:

- Medium-sized pork chops, approximately 3.5 ounces each
- 1 cup of breadcrumbs (Panko brand works well)
- medium-sized eggs
- Pinch of salt and pepper
- ½ tablespoon of mint, either dried and ground; or fresh, rinsed and finely chopped

Directions:

1 Preparing the Ingredients. Cover the Air fryer oven basket with a lining of tin foil, leaving the edges uncovered to allow air to circulate through the basket. Preheat the Air fryer oven to 350 degrees.

2 In a bowl, beat the eggs until fluffy until the yolks and whites are completely combined and set aside.

3 In a separate bowl, combine the crumbs, mint, salt, and pepper and set aside. One at a time, dip each raw pork chop into the dry ingredient bowl, coat all sides, then dip it into the wet ingredient bowl, then dip it back into the dry ingredients. This double layer will ensure cooler air. Place the breaded pork chops on the oven rack,

in a single flat layer. Place the air fryer rack on the middle shelf of the fryer.

4 Air fry. Set the Air Fryer timer to 15 minutes. After 15 minutes the Air Fryer oven will turn off and the pork should cook in the middle and the bread layer should start to brown. Using tweezers, flip each piece of meat over to secure a full pair of pants. Return the fryer to 320 degrees for 15 minutes.

5 After 15 minutes, when the fryer is off, remove the fried pork chops with tongs and place in a source. Eat as fresh as you can, and enjoy!

Nutrition:

Calories: 213;

Fat: 9g;

Protein: 12g;

Fiber: 3g

242. Fried Chicken Livers

Difficulty: Easy

Preparation Time: 5 Minutes

Cooking Time: 10 Minutes

Servings: 4

Ingredients:

- 1 pound chicken livers
- 1 cup flour
- 1/2 cup cornmeal
- teaspoons your favorite seasoning blend
- eggs
- tablespoons milk

Directions:

1 Preparing the Ingredients. Clean and rinse the livers, pat dry.

2 Beat eggs in a shallow bowl and mix in milk.

3 In another bowl combine flour, cornmeal, and seasoning, mixing until even.

4 Dip the livers in the egg mix, then toss them in the flour mix.

5 Air Frying. Air-fry at 375 degrees for 10 minutes using your Air fryer oven. Toss at least once halfway through.

Nutrition:

Calories: 409;

Fat: 11g;

Protein: 36g;

Fiber: 2g

243. Crispy Southern Fried Chicken

Difficulty: Easy

Preparation Time: 10 Minutes

Cooking Time: 25 Minutes

Servings: 4

Ingredients:

- 1 tsp. cayenne pepper
- tbsp. mustard powder
- tbsp. oregano
- tbsp. thyme
- tbsp. coconut milk

- 1 beaten egg
- ¼ C. cauliflower
- ¼ C. gluten-free oats
- chicken drumsticks

Directions:

1. Preparing the Ingredients. Ensure the Air fryer oven is preheated to 350 degrees.
2. Lay out chicken and season with pepper and salt on all sides.
3. Add all other ingredients to a blender, blending till a smooth-like breadcrumb mixture is created. Place in a bowl and add a beaten egg to another bowl.
4. Dip chicken into breadcrumbs, then into the egg, and breadcrumbs once more. Air Frying. Place coated drumsticks into the Air fryer oven. Set temperature to 350°F, and set time to 20 minutes and cook 20 minutes. Bump up the temperature to 390 degrees and cook another 5 minutes till crispy.

Nutrition:

Calories: 504; Fat: 18g; Protein: 35g; Sugar: 5g

244. Tex-Mex Turkey Burgers

Difficulty: Easy

Preparation Time: 10 Minutes

Cooking Time: 15 Minutes

Servings: 4

Ingredients:

- 1/3 cup finely crushed corn tortilla chips
- 1 egg, beaten
- ¼ cup salsa
- 1/3 cup shredded pepper Jack cheese
- Pinch salt
- Freshly ground black pepper
- 1 pound ground turkey
- 1 tablespoon olive oil
- 1 teaspoon paprika

Directions:

1. Preparing the Ingredients. In a small bowl, combine the tortilla chips, egg, salsa, cheese, salt, pepper, and mix well.
2. Add the turkey and mix gently but thoroughly with clean hands.
3. Form the meat mixture into patties about ½ inch thick. Make an indentation in the center of each patty with your thumb, so the burgers don't puff up while cooking.
4. Brush the patties on each sides with the olive oil and sprinkle with paprika.
5. Air Frying. Put in the Oven rack/basket. Place the tray rack on the middle-shelf of the Air fryer oven. Grill for 14 to 16 minutes or until the meat registers at least 165°F.

Nutrition:

Calories: 354;

Fat: 21g;

Protein: 36g;

Fiber: 2g

245. Air Fryer Turkey Breast

Difficulty: Easy

Preparation Time: 5 Minutes

Cooking Time: 60 Minutes

Servings: 6

Ingredients:

- Pepper and salt
- 1 oven-ready turkey breast
- Turkey seasonings of choice

Directions:

1 Preparing the Ingredients. Preheat the Air fryer oven to 350 degrees.

2 Season turkey with pepper, salt, and other desired seasonings.

3 Place turkey in the Oven rack/basket. Place the tray Rack on the middle-shelf of the Air fryer oven.

4 Air Frying. Set temperature to 350°F, and set time to 60 minutes. Cook 60 minutes. The meat should be at 165 degrees when done.

5 Allow to rest 10-15 minutes before slicing. Enjoy!

Nutrition:

Calories: 212;

Fat: 12g;

Protein: 24g;

Sugar: 0g

246. Mustard Chicken Tenders

Difficulty: Medium

Preparation Time: 5 Minutes

Cooking Time: 20 Minutes

Servings: 4

Ingredients:

- ½ C. coconut flour
- 1 tbsp. spicy brown mustard
- beaten eggs
- 1 pound of chicken tenders

Directions:

1 Preparing the Ingredients. Season tenders with pepper and salt.

2 Place a thin layer of mustard onto tenders and then dredge in flour and dip in egg.

3 Air Frying. Add to the Air fryer oven, set temperature to 390°F, and set time to 20 minutes.

Nutrition:

Calories: 403; Fat: 20g; Protein: 22g; Sugar: 4g

247. Chicken Nuggets

Difficulty: Medium

Preparation Time: 10 Minutes

Cooking Time: 20 Minutes

Servings: 4

Ingredients:

- 1 pound boneless, skinless chicken breasts
- chicken seasoning or rub

- salt
- pepper
- eggs
- 1 tablespoons bread crumbs
- 1 tablespoons panko bread crumbs
- cooking oil

Directions:

1 Preparation of ingredients. Cut the chicken breasts into 1-inch pieces.

2 In a large bowl, add together the chicken pieces with the chicken seasoning, salt, and pepper.

3 In a small bowl, beat the eggs. In another bowl, combine breadcrumbs and countertop.

4 Dip the chicken pieces in the eggs and then the breadcrumbs.

5 Place the pepitas in the deep fryer. Don't overdo the basket. Cook in batches. Drizzle the seeds with cooking oil.

6 Air Frying. Cook for 4 minutes. Open the Air fryer oven and shake the basket. Set temperature to 360°F. Cook for an additional 4 minutes. Remove the cooked nuggets from the Air fryer oven, repeat steps 5 and 6 for the remaining chicken nuggets. Cool before serving.

Nutrition:

Calories: 206; Fat: 5g;

Protein: 31g; Fiber: 1g

248. Cheesy Chicken Fritters

Difficulty: Medium

Preparation Time: 5 Minutes

Cooking Time: 20 Minutes

Servings: 17

Ingredients:

- Chicken Fritters:
- ½ tsp. salt
- 1/8 tsp. pepper
- 1 ½ tbsp. fresh dill
- 1 1/3 C. shredded mozzarella cheese
- 1/3 C. coconut flour
- 1/3 C. vegan mayo
- eggs
- 1 ½ pounds chicken breasts
- Garlic Dip:
- 1/8 tsp. pepper
- ¼ tsp. salt
- ½ tbsp. lemon juice
- 1 pressed garlic cloves
- 1/3 C. vegan mayo

Directions:

1 Preparing the Ingredients. Slice chicken breasts into 1/3" pieces and place in a bowl. Add all remaining fritter ingredients to the bowl and stir well. Cover and chill 2 hours or overnight.

2 Ensure your air fryer is preheated to 350 degrees. Spray basket with a bit of olive oil.

3. Air Frying. Add marinated chicken to the Air fryer oven. Set temperature to 350°F, set time to 20 minutes and cook 20 minutes, making sure to turn halfway through the cooking process.
4. To make the dipping sauce, combine all the dip ingredients until smooth.

Nutrition:

Calories: 467;

Fat: 27g;

Protein: 21g;

Sugar: 3g

249. Air Fryer Chicken Parmesan

Difficulty: Medium

Preparation Time: 5 Minutes

Cooking Time: 9 Minutes

Servings: 4

Ingredients:

- ½ C. keto marinara
- 1 tbsp. mozzarella cheese
- 1 tbsp. melted ghee
- 1 tbsp. grated parmesan cheese
- 1 tbsp. gluten-free seasoned breadcrumbs
- 8-ounce chicken breasts

Directions:

1. Preparing the Ingredients. Ensure air fryer is preheated to 360 degrees. Spray the basket with olive oil.
2. Mix parmesan cheese and breadcrumbs together. Melt ghee.
3. Brush melted ghee onto the chicken and dip into breadcrumb mixture.
4. Place coated chicken in the air fryer and top with olive oil.
5. Air Frying. Set temperature to 360°F, and set time to 6 minutes. Cook 2 breasts for 6 minutes and top each breast with a tablespoon of sauce and 1½ tablespoons of mozzarella cheese. Cook another 3 minutes to melt cheese.
6. Keep cooked pieces warm as you repeat the process with remaining breasts.

Nutrition:

Calories: 251;

Fat: 10g;

Protein: 31g;

Sugar: 0g

250. Ricotta and Parsley Stuffed Turkey Breasts

Difficulty: Medium

Preparation Time: 5 Minutes

Cooking Time: 25 Minutes

Servings: 4

Ingredients:

- 1 turkey breast, quartered
- 1 cup Ricotta cheese
- 1/4 cup fresh Italian parsley, chopped
- 1 teaspoon garlic powder

- 1/2 teaspoon cumin powder
- 1 egg, beaten
- 1 teaspoon paprika
- Salt and ground black pepper, to taste
- Crushed tortilla chips
- 1 ½ tablespoons extra-virgin olive oil

Directions:

1. Preparing the Ingredients. Firstly, flatten out each piece of turkey breast with a rolling pin. Prepare three mixing bowls.
2. In a shallow bowl, combine Ricotta cheese with the parsley, garlic powder, and cumin powder.
3. Place the Ricotta/parsley mixture in the middle of each piece. Repeat with the remaining pieces of the turkey breast and roll them up.
4. In another shallow bowl, whisk the egg together with paprika. In the third shallow bowl, combine the salt, pepper, and crushed tortilla chips.
5. Dip each roll in the whisked egg, then, roll them over the tortilla chips mixture.
6. Transfer prepared rolls to the Oven rack/basket. Drizzle olive oil over all. Place the tray Rack on the middle-shelf of the Air fryer oven.
7. Air Frying. Cook for 25 minutes at 350 degrees F, working in batches. Serve warm, garnished with some extra parsley, if desired.

Nutrition:

Calories: 509;

Fat: 23g;

Protein: 26g;

Fiber: 5g

CHAPTER 13:

Vegetarian And Vegan Recipes

251. Sweet Potato Casserole

Preparation Time: minutes

Cooking Time: minutes

Servings: 4

Cooking Time: 15 minutes

Servings: 4

Ingredients

2 c. sweet potatoes

¼ c. melted butter

1½ tbsp. milk

¼ c. honey

vanilla

1 large egg

¼ c. brown sugar

¼ c. wheat flour

2 tbsp. butter

½ c. chopped pecans

Cooking spray

Directions

Spray baking sheet with cooking spray.

In a large mixing bowl, combine milk, honey, sweet potatoes, vanilla, melted butter, and egg. Mix well.

In another mixing bowl, combine brown sugar and flour. Cut in 3 tablespoons butter till crumbly. Add pecans and mix well.

Sprinkle the mixture over sweet potatoes.

Place on 1-inch rack and cook for 25-30 minutes at 350°C (High) or until golden brown.

Serve Immediately.

Nutrition:

Calories: 310

Total Fat: 13g

Carbs: 49g

Protein: 3g

252. Fruit and Vegetable Skewers

Preparation Time: 60 minutes

Cooking Time: 20 minutes

Servings: 4

Ingredients

4 tbsp virgin olive oil

3 tbsp. lemon juice

1 garlic clove, minced

2 tbsp. chopped parsley

½ tsp. salt

½ tsp. black pepper

1 sliced zucchini

1 sliced yellow squash

½ red bell pepper

½ c. cherry tomatoes

½ c. pineapple chunks

4 wooden skewers

Directions

In a large mixing bowl combine olive oil, garlic, parsley, lemon juice, pepper, and salt. Pour into large resalable plastic bag. Add zucchini, squash, bell pepper, and tomatoes. Seal bag, shake to coat vegetables, and place in refrigerator for a minimum of 1 hour.

Remove vegetables from marinade and thread onto skewers, along with pineapple, alternating among each item.

Line bottom of NuWave Oven with foil for easier clean-up.

Place skewers on the 4-inch rack. Cook on High Power (350°C) for 8 minutes.

Flip skewers over and cook for another 6-8 minutes until veggies are desired level of doneness.

Remove from NuWave Oven, transfer to a plate, and serve.

Nutrition:

Calories: 173 Total Fat: 2.8 g

Total carbs: 36.5g Protein: 5g

253. Roasted Sweet Potatoes with Rosemary

Preparation Time: 15 minutes

Cooking Time: 12 minutes

Servings: 4

Ingredients

1 ½ pound sweet potatoes, cubed

1 tsp. olive oil

1 dash chopped rosemary

1 dash lemon juice

Directions

In a bowl, toss sweet potatoes with oil. Evenly spread on the 10-inch baking sheet, sprinkle with rosemary. Place on 1-inch rack and back on High power (350 degrees F) for 12 minutes. Flip sweet potatoes over and cook an additional 10 minutes.

Drizzle with lemon juice and serve.

Nutrition:

Calories: 114

Total fat: 0g

Carbs: 27g

Protein: 2g

254. Tangy Roasted Broccoli with Garlic

Preparation Time: 10 minutes

Cooking Time: 15 minutes

Servings: 4

Ingredients

1 broccoli head

3 garlic cloves, minced

2 tsp. virgin olive oil

1 tsp. sea salt

½ tsp. black pepper

½ tsp. lemon juice

Directions

In a mixing bowl, add oil, salt, garlic and black pepper. Add broccoli. Mix to coat. Evenly scatter broccoli on the 10-inch baking sheet.

Place on1-inch rack and roast on High power (350 degrees F) for about 10 minutes. Flip florets and cook another 5-7 minutes or until fork tender.

Plate and drizzle lemon juice. Serve at once.

Nutrition:

Calories: 141

Carbs: 10g

Fat: 10 g

Protein: 5g

255. Roasted Carrots with Garlic

Preparation Time: 10 minutes

Cooking Time: 20 minutes

Servings: 2

Ingredients

3 tbsp. olive oil

2 minced garlic cloves

Sea salt, to taste

1 pound baby carrots

Directions

In a medium bowl, mix carrots with olive oil, salt and garlic. Spread carrots in single layer on parchment or foil-lined baking sheet.

Place on 1-inch rack and cook on High power (350 F) for 15-20 minutes until carrots are tender.

Nutrition:

Calories: 95

Total Fat: 6.9g

Total carbs: 7.6g

Protein: 1g

256. Savory Roasted Balsamic Vegetables

Preparation Time: 10 minutes

Cooking Time: 30 minutes

Servings: 4

Ingredients

1½ c. cubed butternut squash

1 c. chopped broccoli florets

½ chopped red onion

1 chopped zucchini

1 minced garlic clove

2 tbsp. virgin olive oil

1½ tsp. rosemary

A pinch of salt, to taste

1 tbsp. balsamic vinegar

Directions

In a mixing bowl, add oil, rosemary, vinegar, pepper, and salt; mix to blend. Mix in the vegetables, mix to coat evenly.

Evenly spread on a parchment-lined baking sheet.

Place on 1-inch rack and cook on High power (350 degrees F) for about 15 minutes. Flip vegetables and cook for another 15 minutes or until squash is just softened.

Nutrition:

Calories: 148

Total Fat: 4.6g

Total carbs: 25g

Protein: 7g

257. Baked Macaroni and Cheese

Preparation Time: 10 minutes

Cooking Time: 25 minutes

Servings: 4

Ingredients

½ pound Cheddar cheese, shredded

4 tbsp. butter

2 eggs

1 tsp. Dijon mustard

12 oz. evaporated milk

1 pound elbow macaroni

Salt and black pepper to taste

½ c. breadcrumbs

Directions

Cook macaroni according to package directions.

Spray casserole dish with cooking spray.

Add all ingredients except for bread crumbs to a casserole dish and mix well to combine. Sprinkle with breadcrumbs.

Cover with foil and place pan on 1-inch rack. Bake on High (350 degrees F) for 15-20 minutes. Remove the foil then cook for another 5-10 minutes or until golden brown.

Nutrition:

Calories: 480

Total Fat: 19g

Carbs: 31g

Protein: 24g

258. Curried Zucchini Chips

Preparation Time: 10 minutes

Cooking Time: 24 minutes

Servings: 2

Ingredients

1 medium sliced zucchini

1 tbsp. virgin olive oil

⅛ tsp. garlic powder

¼ tsp. curry powder

⅛ tsp. salt

Directions

Lightly grease paper-lined baking sheet. Arrange zucchini slices in one layer on the baking sheet. Sprinkle olive oil and dust with curry powder, salt, and garlic powder.

Place baking sheet on 1-inch rack and bake on High power (350 degrees F) for 12 minutes. Flip zucchini over and cook for another 10 minutes or till very crisp. Cool and store in airtight container

Nutrition:

Calories: 152 Total carbs: 17g Total Fat: 3g

Protein: 2g

259. Vegan Pear and Cranberry Cake

Preparation Time: 5 minutes

Cooking Time: 45 minutes

Servings: 4-6

Ingredients

Dry Ingredients

1 1/4 cup whole wheat pastry flour

1/8 teaspoon sea salt

1/2 teaspoon baking powder

1/2 teaspoon baking soda

1/2 teaspoon ground cardamom

Wet Ingredients

1/2 cup unsweetened nondairy milk

2 tablespoons coconut oil

2 tablespoons ground flax seeds

1/4 cup agave

1 1/2 cups water

Mix-Ins

1/2 cup chopped cranberries

1 cup chopped pear

Directions

Grease a Bundt pan; set aside.

In a mixing, mix all dry ingredients together. In another bowl, mix all wet ingredients; whisk the wet ingredients into the dry until smooth. Fold in the add-ins and spread the mixture into the pan; cover with foil. Place pan in your air fryer toast oven and add water in the bottom and bake at 370 degrees F for 35 minutes. When done, use a toothpick to check for doneness. Of it comes out clean, then the cake is ready, if not, bake for 5-10 more minutes, checking frequently to avoid burning. Remove the cake and let stand for 10 minutes before transferring from the pan. Enjoy!

Nutrition. Calories: 309 kcal, Carbs: 14.7 g, Fat: 27 g, Protein: 22.6 g.

260. Air fryer toast oven Steamed Broccoli

Preparation Time: 8 minutes

Cooking Time: 3 minutes

Servings: 2

Ingredients

1 pound broccoli florets

1½ cups water

Salt and pepper to taste

I tsp. extra virgin olive oil

Directions

Add water to the bottom of your air fryer toast oven and set the basket on top.

Toss the broccoli florets with, salt pepper and olive oil until evenly combined then transfer to the basket of your air fryer toast oven.

Cook at 350 degrees for 5 minutes.

Remove the basket and serve the broccoli.

Nutrition:

Calories: 160 kcal

Carbs: 6.1 g

Fat: 12 g

Protein: 13 g.

Conclusion

Hopefully, after going through this book and trying out a couple of recipes, you will understand the flexibility and utility of the Breville smart air fryers. It is undoubtedly a multipurpose kitchen appliance that is highly recommended to everybody. It presents one with a palatable atmosphere to enjoy fried foods that are delicious but healthy, cheaper, and more convenient. The use of this kitchen appliance ensures that the making of some of your favorite snacks and meals will be carried out in a stress-free manner without hassling around, which invariably legitimizes its worth and gives you value for your money.

This book will be your all-time guide to understand the basics of the Breville smart air fryer because, with all the recipes mentioned in the book, you are rest assured that it will be something that you and the rest of the people around the world will enjoy for the rest of your lives. You will be able to prepare delicious and flavorsome meals that will be easy to carry out but tasty and healthy.

However, you should never limit yourself to the recipes solely mentioned in this cookbook, go on and try new things! Explore new recipes! Experiment with different ingredients, seasonings, and different methods! Create some new recipes and keep your mind open. By so doing, you will be able to get the best out of your Breville smart air fryer oven.

We are so glad you leaped this healthier cooking format with us!

The air fryer truly is not a gadget that should stay on the shelf. Instead, take it out and give it a whirl when you are whipping up one of your tried-and-true recipes, or if you are starting to get your feet wet with the air frying method.

Regardless of appliances, recipes, or dietary concerns, we hope you have fun in your kitchen. Between food preparation, cooking time, and then the cleanup, a lot of time is spent in this one room, so it should be as fun as possible.

This is just the start. There are no limits to working with the Breville smart air fryer, and we will explore some more recipes. In addition to all the great options that we talked about before, you will find that there are tasty desserts that can those sweet teeth in no time, and some great sauces and dressing to always be in control over the foods you eat. There are just so many options to choose from that it won't take long before you find a whole bunch of recipes to use, and before you start to wonder why you didn't get the Breville smart air fryer so much sooner. There are so many things to admire about the air fryer, and it becomes an even better tool to use when you have the right recipes in place and can use them. And there are so many fantastic recipes that work well in the air fryer and can get dinner on the table in no time. We are pleased that you pursue this Breville smart Air Fryer oven cookbook. Happy, healthy eating!

7 days Omnivorous Breville Air Fryer Oven Meal Plan

Days	Breakfast	Lunch	Dinner	vegetables
Days 1	Breakfast Ham Omelet	Rolled Salmon Sandwich	Cheeseburger Egg Rolls	Crusted scallops
Days 2	Breakfast Chicken Strips	Balsamic Roasted Chicken	Air Fried Grilled Steak	Lobster tails with white wine sauce
Days 3	Chicken & Zucchini Omelet	Chicken Capers Sandwich	Juicy Cheeseburgers	Broiled lobster tails
Days 4	Potatoes with Bacon	Easy Prosciutto Grilled Cheese	Spicy Thai Beef Stir-Fry	Sheet pan seafood bake
Days 5	Shrimp Sandwiches	Herb-Roasted Chicken Tenders	Beef Brisket Recipe from Texas	Lobster tails with lemon butter
Days 6	Tuna Sandwiches	Moroccan Pork Kebabs	Copycat Taco Bell Crunch Wraps	Buttery scallops
Days 7	Almond Crust Chicken	Pecan Crunch Catfish and Asparagus	Steak and Mushroom Gravy	Broiled lobster tails

7 days Vegetarian Breville Air Fryer Oven Meal Plan

Days	Breakfast	Lunch	Dinner	vegetables
Days 1	Citrus Blueberry Muffins	Roasted Beet Salad with Oranges & Beet Greens	Sweet Potato Casserole	Fruity crumble
Days 2	PB &J Donuts	Vegetable Egg Rolls	Fruit and Vegetable Skewers	Cherry clafoutis
Days 3	Breakfast Baked Apple	Spinach Quiche	Roasted Sweet Potatoes with Rosemary	Apple bread pudding
Days 4	Sunny Side up Egg Tarts	Lentils Fritters	Tangy Roasted Broccoli with Garlic	Masala Cashew
Days 5	Healthy Spinach Scramble	Corn Casserole	Roasted Carrots with Garlic	Donuts pudding
Days 6	Bread Rolls	Air Fried Mushroom Frittata	Savory Roasted Balsamic Vegetables	Buttery scallops
Days 7	Walnuts Pear Oatmeal	Jumbo Stuffed Mushrooms	Baked Macaroni and Cheese	Divided Balsamic Mustard Greens

Index

D

E

F

R

S

T

V

W

Y

Z

CPSIA information can be obtained
at www.ICGtesting.com
Printed in the USA
LVHW060808120221
679113LV00023B/776

9 781801 327862